中医经典译丛

Chinese-English Translation of Traditional Chinese Medicine Classics

# 食 疗 本 草

## Materia Medica for Dietotherapy

（汉英对照）

原　著　〔唐〕孟　诜　〔唐〕张　鼎

主　译　孙　慧

副主译　赵　栋　周　茜

译　者　王 丽 君　邱　冬　周　茜

　　　　赵　栋　孙　慧

本书为山东中医药大学"中医英译及中医文化对外传播研究"科研创新团队项目资助成果、山东中医药大学英语专业学科建设资助成果

U0396095

苏州大学出版社

**图书在版编目（CIP）数据**

食疗本草：汉英对照／（唐）孟诜，（唐）张鼎原著：
孙慧主译. —苏州：苏州大学出版社，2020.4
（中医经典译丛）
书名原文：Materia Medica for Dietotherapy
ISBN 978-7-5672-2950-1

Ⅰ.①食… Ⅱ.①孟… ②张… ③孙… Ⅲ.①食物本
草-中国-唐代-汉、英 Ⅳ.①R281.5

中国版本图书馆 CIP 数据核字（2019）第 204897 号

书　　名：食疗本草 SHI LIAO BEN CAO
　　　　　Materia Medica for Dietotherapy
　　　　　（汉英对照）

原　　著：〔唐〕孟　诜　〔唐〕张　鼎
主　　译：孙　慧
责任编辑：汤定军
策划编辑：汤定军
装帧设计：刘　俊

出版发行：苏州大学出版社（Soochow University Press）
社　　址：苏州市十梓街 1 号　邮编：215006
印　　装：虎彩印艺股份有限公司
网　　址：www. sudapress. com
邮　　箱：sdcbs@ suda. edu. cn
邮购热线：0512-67480030
销售热线：0512-67481020

开　　本：700mm×1 000mm　1/16　印张：16　字数：271 千
版　　次：2020 年 4 月第 1 版
印　　次：2020 年 4 月第 1 次印刷
书　　号：ISBN 978-7-5672-2950-1
定　　价：68.00 元

凡购本社图书发现印装错误，请与本社联系调换。服务热线：0512-67481020

# 翻译说明

1. 本次所译的《食疗本草》以宋代唐慎微《证类本草》中所辑录的《食疗本草》内容为基础,并参考了敦煌残卷和《医心方》中引录的条文以及多个《食疗本草》的通行本。

2. 为了更准确地表达和传递《食疗本草》的内容,本书的本草采用中文原文、中文注释、英文译文、英文注释进行编排。个别中药名经多方考证仍无法确定其拉丁名称,翻译成拉丁文的时候,采取 Materia Medica 加音译的方法,如"船底苔"译为 Materia Medica Chuanditai。

3. 本草名称的翻译采取"四保险"的翻译方法,即每个本草名称均按拼音、汉字、英文和拉丁文的方式进行翻译,如"萹竹"译为 Bianzhu〔萹竹,common knotgrass herb,Herba Polygoni Avicularis〕。

4. 本草名称如果是三个字及以下,其音译合并在一起;如果是四个字及以上,根据文义将其音译分开,便于阅读,如"鹅不食草"音译为 Ebushi Cao。

5. 古籍名称采用音译的方法翻译,括号中附以中文和英文翻译,音译中的每个字独立音译。如《古文尚书》译为 *Gu Wen Shang Shu*〔《古文尚书》,*The Chinese Ancient Classic*〕。

6. 原《食疗本草》卷中条目为动物制品入药,根据《中华人民共和国野生动物保护法》,其中涉及的珍稀野生动物及制品本版不予保留,如犀角、虎、豺等条目。

7. 书中出现的繁体字、异体字根据现行出版规范改为简体字、通行字。中文版原文中有些语言文字与现行出版编辑规范要求不一致的地方,遵从原文。书中涉及的计量单位采用音译方法,基本形式和公制换算如下:

| 传统计量单位 | 公制换算 | 音译形式 |
| --- | --- | --- |
| 尺 | 0.3333333 米 | Chi |
| 寸 | 0.0333333 米 | Cun |
| 丈 | 3.3333333 米 | Zhang |
| 匕 | 2~3 克 | Bi |
| 合 | 0.1 升 | Ge |

# Translation Specification

1. The translation of *Materia Medica for Dietotherapy* is based on the content of *Materia Medica for Dietotherapy* compiled in *Zheng Lei Ben Cao* [《证类本草》, *Materia Medica Arranged According to Pattern*] by Tang Shenwei in the Song Dynasty, and refers to some content in Dunhuang fragments, some formulas in *Yi Xin Fang* [《医心方》, *Formulary from the Heart of Physicians*], as well as several current editions.

2. For more accurate expression and transmission of the content of *Materia Medica for Dietotherapy*, the Chinese-English edition is arranged as follows: Chinese text, Chinese notes, English translation and English notes. Some herbs, even after textual researches, can not locate their Latin names in equivalent, so their Latin translation is presented as "Materia Medica" plus Pinyin. For instance, the Latin translation of "船底苔" is "Materia Medica Chuanditai".

3. As to the translation of herbal names, the "Four Assurance Method" is adopted, namely, every herbal name is translated in the way that its four forms are listed in the sequence of Pinyin, Chinese character, English and Latin. For instance, "萹竹" is translated as Bianzhu [萹竹, common knotgrass herb, Herba Polygoni Avicularis].

4. If a herbal name has three or less than three Chinese characters, its transliteration of Pinyin is put together; if it has four or more than four Chinese characters, its transliteration of Pinyin is divided into two parts according to its literal meaning for the convenience of easy reading. For instance, the transliteration of "鹅不食草" is "Ebushi Cao".

5. The names of ancient works are transliterated with their Chinese names and English versions in brackets, every Chinese character being transliterated

separately. For instance,《古文尚书》is transliterated as *Gu Wen Shang Shu* [《古文尚书》, *The Chinese Ancient Classic*].

6. According to the *Law of the People's Republic of China on the Protection of Wildlife*, rare wild animals and their related products involved in the Chinese version of the original text are not retained in this Chinese-English edition, such as rhino horn, tiger, jackal, etc.

7. The traditional Chinese characters and variant Chinese characters in the Chinese version of the original text are changed into the simplified and current Chinese characters in this Chinese-English edition according to the current publishing standards. Some expressions in the Chinese version of the original text, inconsistent with the requirements of the current publication specifications, are retained the style of the original text. The names of units of measurement in this book are transliterated by Pinyin, the examples of them and metric conversion refer to the table below:

| Traditional Unit | Metric Conversion | Pinyin |
|:---:|:---:|:---:|
| 尺 | 0. 3333333 meter | Chi |
| 寸 | 0. 0333333 meter | Cun |
| 丈 | 3. 3333333 meters | Zhang |
| 匕 | 2 ~ 3 grams | Bi |
| 合 | 0. 1 litre | Ge |

# 目 录

# Contents

## Volume 1

# Contents

## Volume 2

# Contents

# Contents

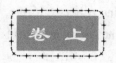

# Volume 1

## 1. 盐

（一）蠷螋尿疮<sup>[1]</sup>：盐三升<sup>[2]</sup>，水一斗<sup>[3]</sup>，煮取六升。以绵浸汤，淹疮上。

（二）又，治一切气及脚气<sup>[4]</sup>：取盐三升，蒸，候热分裹，近壁，脚踏之，令脚心热。

（三）又，和槐白皮蒸用，亦治脚气。夜夜与之良。

（四）又，以皂荚两梃，盐半两<sup>[5]</sup>，同烧令通赤，细研。夜夜用揩齿。一月后，有动者齿及血蜃齿，并瘥，其齿牢固。

**【注释】**

［1］蠷（qú）螋（sōu）尿疮：病症名，疮内有白色浆液，疼痛剧烈，并伴有发热等症状。

［2］升：古代的计量单位，唐代1升约合今制0.6升。

［3］斗：古代的计量单位，1斗约合10升，唐代1斗约合今制6升。

［4］脚气：病症名，以腿脚麻木、酸痛、无力或挛急、肿胀为主要特征。

［5］两：古代的计量单位，唐代以大两为主，1大两约合今制40克。

### 1. Yan ［盐, salt, Sal］

For anisolobis sting<sup>[1]</sup>: Boil 3 Sheng<sup>[2]</sup> of Yan ［盐, salt, Sal］ with 1 Dou<sup>[3]</sup> of water, then get 6 Sheng of salt water, soak a piece of cotton cloth in the water and apply the cloth to the sting.

For all diseases caused by qi as the well as the weak foot<sup>[4]</sup>: steam 3 Sheng of salt, wrap it hot in different parcels and let the patients stand against the wall and tread on the parcels until their feet are warm.

It is quite effective in treating the weak foot by steaming it with Huaibaipi ［槐白皮, sophora root bark, Sophorae Cortex Radicis］ and using it every night.

Burn half a Liang[5] of salt with two Zaojia [皂荚, Chinese honey locust, Gleditsia sinensis Lam.] until they are red, grind them finely into powder and rub teeth with the powder every night for one month. Loose teeth will then be tightened, and bleeding gums and dental caries will be cured.

【Notes】

[1] anisolobis sting: It is a disease characterized by white serum in the sores, severe pain and fever.

[2] Sheng: A unit of capacity in ancient times. 1 Sheng in the Tang Dynasty is roughly equivalent to 0.6 Sheng today.

[3] Dou: A unit of capacity in ancient times. 1 Dou in the Tang Dynasty is roughly equivalent to 6 Sheng today, and nowadays 1 Dou is equivalent to 10 Sheng.

[4] weak foot: It is a disease characterized by numbness, ache and weakness, or spasm and swelling of the legs and feet.

[5] Liang: A unit of capacity in ancient times. 1 Liang in the Tang Dynasty is roughly equivalent to 40 grams today.

## 2. 石 燕

(一) 在乳穴石洞中者,冬月采之,堪食。余月采者只堪治病,不堪食也。食如常法。

(二) 又,治法:取石燕二十枚,和五味炒令熟,以酒一斗,浸三日,即每夜卧时饮一两盏[1],随性(多少)也。甚能补益,能吃食,令人健力也。

【注释】

[1] 盏:一种古代的酒器,一盏大约相当于如今的一杯。

### 2. Shiyan [石燕, spirifer fossil, Spiriferae Fossilia]

Shiyan [石燕, spirifer fossil, Spiriferae Fossilia], collected in stalactite caves in the eleventh lunar month, is edible. It can be used only for treating diseases, but not for eating if collected in the remaining months. The way of eating it is the same as that of common food.

Method of treatment: Fry twenty Shiyan with flavorings, soak them in 1 Dou of liquor for three days and take 1 or 2 Zhan[1] of the liquor every night before sleep, but never drink too much. It can be used for tonifying and replenishing, increasing appetite and making people stronger.

**【Note】**

[1] Zhan: A unit of capacity in ancient times. 1 Zhan is roughly equivalent to 1 cup today.

# 3. 黄 精

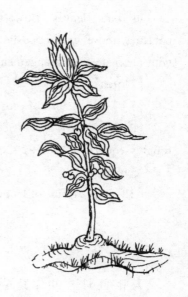

（一）饵黄精,能老不饥。其法:可取瓮子去底,釜上安置令得,所盛黄精令满。密盖,蒸之。令气溜,即暴之。第二遍蒸之亦如此。九蒸九暴。凡生时有一硕[1],熟有三、四斗。蒸之若生,则刺人咽喉;暴使干,不尔朽坏。

（二）其生者,若初服,只可一寸[2]半,渐渐增之。十日不食,能长服之,止三尺[3]五寸。服三百日后,尽见鬼神。饵必升天。

（三）根、叶、花、实,皆可食之。但相对者是,不对者名偏精。

**【注释】**

[1] 硕:古代的计量单位,10 斗为 1 "石"（dàn）。

[2] 寸:古代的计量单位,唐代 1 寸约合今制 0.92 市寸。

[3] 尺:古代的计量单位,1 尺相当于 10 寸。

### 3. Huangjing［黄精, solomonseal rhizome, Rhizoma Polygonati］

Taking Huangjing［黄精, solomonseal rhizome, Rhizoma Polygonati］can prevent aging and tolerate hunger. The procedures: Remove the base of an earthen jar, put the jar in the pot, fill it full with Huangjing, seal it and steam Huangjing until the vapor comes out of it, then take out Huangjing and dry it. The above procedures should be repeated for nine times. 1 Dan[1] of raw Huangjing can be processed into 3 to 4 Dou. It will irritate the throat if not fully steamed, but will not rot easily if dried thoroughly.

It is not allowed to take the raw one longer than one and a half Cun[2] for the first time, but it is allowed to increase gradually to 3 Chi[3] and 5 Cun at most. Taking it for a long time is allowed. Ten-day taking of it can make people live without eating anything else. Three-hundred-day taking of it can make them become mediums. Long-term taking of it can make them become immortals.

Its roots, leaves, flowers and fruits are all edible. More attention should be paid that those with opposite leaf arrangements are called Huangjing, and those with alternate leaf arrangements are called Pianjing(偏精).

【Notes】

[1] Dan：A unit of capacity in ancient times. 1 Dan is equivalent to 10 Dou.

[2] Cun：It is a unit of length in ancient times. 1 Cun in the Tang Dynasty is roughly equivalent to 0.92 Cun today, and 1 Cun nowadays is equivalent to about 3.33 centimeters.

[3] Chi：A unit of length in ancient times. 1 Chi is equivalent to 10 Cun.

# 4. 甘 菊 平

其叶,正月采,可作羹;茎,五月五日采;花,九月九日采。并主头风[1]目眩、泪出,去烦热,利五藏[2]。野生苦菊不堪用。

【注释】

[1] 头风:一种以慢性阵发性风头痛为主要临床表现的疾病。

[2] 五藏:心、肝、脾、肾、肺的合称。藏同"脏"。

## 4. Ganju [甘菊, chrysanthemum, Chrysanthemi Flos] *mild*

Its leaves, collected in the first lunar month, can be made into thick soup. Its stalks can be collected on the 5th of the fifth lunar month, and its flowers on the 9th of the ninth lunar month. It can mainly treat head wind[1], dizzy vision and spontaneous tearing, eliminate vexing fever and harmonize the five zang-organs[2].

Wild bitter chrysanthemum（苦菊）cannot be used as medicine.

【Notes】

［1］head wind：It is a chronic headache caused by invasion of wind into the head.

［2］five zang-organs：It is a collective term for the heart, liver, spleen, lung and kidney.

## 5. 天门冬

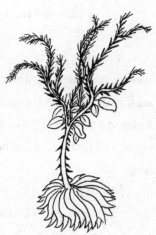

（一）补虚劳[1]，治肺劳[2]，止渴，去热风。可去皮心，入蜜煮之，食后服之。若曝干，入蜜丸尤佳。

（二）亦用洗面，甚佳。

【注释】

［1］虚劳：泛指因阴阳气血亏损而造成的慢性虚症。

［2］肺劳：病症名，因劳损伤肺所致。

### 5. Tianmendong ［天门冬, asparagus root, Radix Asparagi］

It can treat consumptive disease[1] and lung taxation[2], relieve thirst and eliminate wind heat. Peel and core it, boil it with honey and take it after meals. It will be more effective to make honeyed pills after drying it.

It is also quite effective to wash face with it.

【Notes】

［1］consumptive disease：It is a collective term for chronic deficiency diseases due to the consumption of yin, yang, qi and blood.

［2］lung taxation：It is a disease caused by lung damage due to strain.

## 6. 地 黄[1] 微寒

以少蜜煎，或浸食之，或煎汤，或入酒饮，并妙。生则寒，主齿痛，唾血，折伤。叶可以羹。

【注释】

[1] 地黄:玄参科植物地黄的块根。味甘,性寒。有滋阴补肾、养血补血、强心利尿等功效。

### 6. Dihuang[1] [地黄, rehmannia, Radix Rehmanniae] *slightly cold*

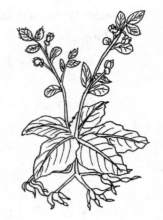

It is effective to decoct it with a small amount of honey, or soak it in water, or decoct it with water, or soak it in liquor. Shengdihuang [生地黄, unprocessed rehmannia root, Radix Rehmanniae Recens] is cold in property and can mainly treat toothache, spitting blood and fracture of the bones and sinews. Its leaves can be used for making thick soup.

【Note】

[1] Dihuang: The root tuber of rehmannia in the family Scrophulariaceae. It is sweet in taste and cold in property. It has the effects of nourishing yin and tonifying the kidney, nourishing and replenishing the blood, strengthening the heart and disinhibiting urine, etc.

# 7. 薯蓣(山药)

治头疼,利丈夫,助阴力。和面作馎饦[1],则微动气,为不能制面毒也。熟煮和蜜,或为汤煎,或为粉,并佳。干之入药更妙也。

【注释】

[1] 馎饦:古代一种水煮的面食。

### 7. Shuyu (Shanyao) [薯蓣(山药), common yam rhizome, Rhizoma Dioscoreae]

It can treat headache and is beneficial to male sexual functions. It will stir qi slightly when kneading the dough with it, boiling the dough into Botuo[1] and eating Botuo, because it cannot disperse the toxin in flour. It is beneficial to health by mixing the boiled one with honey, or decocting it with water, or grinding it into powder. It will be even better for medicinal uses after drying it.

【Note】

[1] Botuo: It is a water-boiled pasta in ancient China.

## 8. 白 蒿 寒

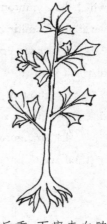

（一）春初此蒿前诸草生。捣汁去热黄[1]及心痛。其叶生授,醋淹之为菹,甚益人。

（二）又,叶干为末,夏日暴水痢[2],以米饮和一匙,空腹服之。

（三）子:主鬼气[3],末和酒服之良。

（四）又,烧淋灰煎,治淋沥[4]疾。

【注释】

[1] 热黄:湿热型黄疸,湿热之邪所致,呈身目俱黄、发热口渴、心烦欲呕、小便黄赤、便秘等症状。

[2] 暴水痢:痢疾,病症名,以大便次数增多、腹痛、里急后重、下痢赤白脓血为主要特征。此处"暴"指突发或急性。

[3] 鬼气:因中了鬼物邪气而引起的疾病。古人认为神志昏乱、言语无度、行动失常等病症的发病原因在于鬼气。

[4] 淋沥:淋证,病症名,主要表现为以小便频急、淋沥不尽、尿道涩痛、小腹拘急、痛引腰腹。

## 8. Baihao［白蒿, sievers wormwood herb, Herba Artemisiae Scopariae］*cold*

It sprouts earlier than other grass-like plants in early spring. Its juice can treat damp-heat jaundice[1] and heart pain. Its fresh leaves, rubbed and pickled into Chinese sauerkraut with vinegar, can nourish the human body.

It can treat acute dysentery[2] in summer by drying its leaves, grinding them into powder, mixing a spoon of powder with rice soup and taking the soup before meals.

Its seeds can mainly treat ghost qi[3]. It will have a good effect when grinding it into powder and taking the powder with liquor.

It can treat stranguria[4] by burning it into ash, filtering the ash with water and making decoction.

【Notes】

［1］damp-heat jaundice：It is a type of jaundice caused by dampness heat, which has symptoms such as yellow discoloration of the skin and sclera, fever, thirst, vexation, vomiting, yellow discoloration of the urine and constipation.

［2］dysentery：It is a disease characterized by abdominal pain, tenesmus, diarrhea with stool containing mucus and blood.

［3］ghost qi：It is a disease caused by ghosts and evil qi. The ancients believed that ghost qi was the cause of the disorder of mind, speech and behavior.

［4］stranguria：It is a disease characterized by micturition, dribbling urine, urethral ache, lower abdominal spasm, abdominal pain and lumbago.

# 9. 决明子 平

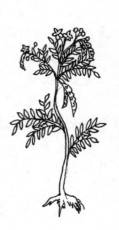

（一）叶：主明目,利五藏,食之甚良。

（二）子：主肝家热毒气,风眼赤泪。每日取一匙,挼去尘埃,空腹水吞之。百日后,夜见物光也。

## 9. Juemingzi ［决明子, cassia seed, Semen Cassiae］ *mild*

Its leaves can improve vision and harmonize the five zang-organs. Eating it is especially beneficial to health.

Its seeds can mainly disperse heat toxin in the liver and treat wind eye and spontaneous tearing. Take a spoon of its seeds, wipe the dust off them and eat them with water every day before meals. In one hundred days, the vision will be improved to see things at night.

## 10．生　姜 温

（一）去痰下气。多食少心智。八九月食，伤神。

（二）除壮热，治转筋，心满。食之除鼻塞，去胸中臭气，通神明。

（三）又，冷痢[1]：取椒烙之为末，共干姜末等分，以醋和面，作小馄饨子，服二七枚。先以水煮，更之饮中重煮。出，停冷吞之。以粥饮下，空腹，日一度作之良。

（四）谨按：止逆，散烦闷，开胃气。又姜屑末和酒服之，除偏风[2]。汁作煎，下一切结实[3]冲胸膈恶气[4]，神验。

（五）又，胃气虚[5]，风热，不能食：姜汁半鸡子壳，生地黄汁少许，蜜一匙头，和水三合[6]，顿服立瘥。

（六）又，皮寒，（姜）性温。

（七）又，姜汁和杏仁汁煎成煎，酒调服，或水调下。善下一切结实冲胸膈。

【注释】

[1] 冷痢：肠虚寒客所致的痢疾。

[2] 偏风：半身不遂。

[3] 结实：饮食等停积于肠胃而引发的腹胀、呕吐、食欲减退、便秘等症状。

[4] 恶气：因气血阻滞而产生瘀浊的一种病理性产物。

[5] 胃气虚：胃的收纳和消化功能虚弱。

[6] 合（gě）：古代的计量单位，10 合相当于 1 升。

## 10. Shengjiang［生姜, rhizome of common ginger, Rhizoma Zingiberis Recens］*warm*

It can direct qi downward and dispel phlegm. Excessive eating of it will damage people's mind. Eating it in the eighth and ninth lunar month is harmful to people's spirit.

It can treat vigorous heat, spasm and heart fullness. Eating it can eliminate nasal congestion, remove foul smell in the chest and invigorate spirit and mentality.

For cold dysentery[1]: Bake Huajiao［花椒, pricklyash peel, Pericarpium

Zanthoxyli], grind it into powder, mix the powder with equal amount of Ganjiang [干姜, dry ginger, Rhizoma Zingiberis] powder, and knead the dough with vinegar, and then make wontons. Boil wontons first in water and then in rice soup, cool them and take them with porridge. It is appropriate to take 14 wontons at a time every morning before meals.

The following is supplemented by Zhang Ding: It can relieve vomitting, disperse vexation and open stomach qi. It can treat hemilateral wind[2] by taking its powder with liquor. It can dispel repletion binds[3] and disperse malign qi[4] towards the chest and diaphragm by decocting its juice and taking the decoction.

For stomach qi deficiency[5], wind heat and loss of appetite: Mix half an egg shell amount of its juice with a little juice of Shengdihuang [生地黄, unprocessed rehmannia root, Radix Rehmanniae Recens], a spoon of honey and 3 Ge[6] of water, take the juice completely at a time and can recover instantly.

It is warm in property, but its skin is cold in property.

It can effectively dispel repletion binds and disperse malign qi towards the chest and diaphragm by mixing its juice with the juice of Xingren [杏仁, bitter apricot seed, Semen Armeniacae Amarum], decocting them and taking the decoction with liquor or water.

【Notes】

[1] cold dysentery: It is a kind of dysentery caused by deficiency cold and gastrointestinal weakness in the stomach and intestine.

[2] hemilateral wind: Hemiplegia.

[3] repletion binds: They refer to pathological changes characterized by abdominal distention, vomiting, impaired appetite and constipation due to food retention in the stomach and intestine.

[4] malign qi: TCM terminology referring to the pathological product of the stasis turbidity due to obstruction of qi and blood.

[5] stomach qi deficiency: It is a pathogenesis which refers to the weak receptive and digestive function of the stomach.

[6] Ge: A unit of capacity in ancient times. 10 spoons are equal to 1 Ge, and 10 Ge are equal to 1 Sheng.

## 11. 苍 耳 温

（一）主中风[1]、伤寒[2]头痛。

（二）又，丁肿[3]困重，生捣苍耳根、叶，和小儿尿绞取汁，冷服一升，日三度，甚验。

（三）拔丁肿根脚。

（四）又，治一切风：取嫩叶一石，切，捣和五升麦蘖，团作块。于蒿、艾中盛二十日，状成曲。取米一斗，炊作饭。看冷暖，入苍耳麦蘖曲，作三大升酿之。封一十四日成熟。取此酒，空心暖服之，神验。封此酒可两重布，不得全密，密则溢出。

（五）又，不可和马肉食。

【注释】

[1] 中风：气血逆乱导致脑脉痹阻或血溢脑脉之外，主要表现为卒暴昏仆、不省人事，或突然口眼㖞斜、半身不遂、言语不利。

[2] 伤寒：感受风寒之邪所引起的外感热病的统称。

[3] 丁肿：疔疮，多发于颜面、四肢，以形小根深、坚硬如钉、肿痛灼热、易于走黄、损筋伤骨为主要特征。

## 11. Cang'er［苍耳, xanthium herb, Xanthii Herba］*warm*

It can mainly treat wind stroke[1], cold damage[2] and headache.

When seriously affected by deep-rooted boil[3], it is particularly effective to mash its fresh roots and leaves, mix them with infant's urine, twist them into juice and take 1 Sheng of the juice, three times a day.

It can remove the root of deep-rooted boil.

For all diseases caused by wind evil: Chop 1 Dan of its fresh leaves, mix them with 5 Sheng of Mainie［麦蘖, germinatedbarley, Fructus Hordei Germinatus］, mash them and knead paste one after another. Place the paste in Qinghao［青蒿, sweet wormwood herb, Herba Artemisiae Annuae］ and Aiye［艾叶, argy wormwood leaf, Folium Artemisiae Argyi］ for twenty days until the paste turns into yeast. Cook 1 Dou of rice, mix the rice with 3 Sheng of the yeast when the temperature is appropriate and make liquor with them. The liquor will be ready for drinking after fourteen days of sealing. It will have a good effect when drinking it warm before meals. The container storing the liquor should be covered with two layers of cloth, but not sealed fully for fear that the liquor will overflow.

It is not advisable to eat it together with Marou〔马肉, horse meat, Equi Caro〕.

【Notes】

〔1〕wind stroke：It refers to the brain vessel obstruction or blood flowing over brain vessel caused by derangement of qi and blood, which is characterized by sudden onset of coma and unconsciousness, or deviated eyes and mouth, hemiplegia and impeded speech.

〔2〕cold damage：It is a collective term for various externally contracted febrile diseases caused by wind cold.

〔3〕deep-rooted boil：It mostly occurs on the face or limbs, which has symptoms such as small but deep-rooted boils as hard as nails, swelling, pain, burning heat, running yellow and damage of the sinews and bones.

# 12. 葛 根

蒸食之,消酒毒。其粉亦甚妙。

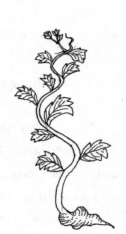

## 12. Gegen〔葛根, kudzuvine root, Radix Puerariae〕

Steaming and eating it can resolve liquor toxin. Its powder is also particularly effective.

# 13. 栝蒌(瓜蒌)

(一) 子:下乳汁。

(二) 又,治痈肿[1]:栝楼根苦酒中熬燥,捣筛之。苦酒和,涂纸上,摊贴。服金石[2]人宜用。

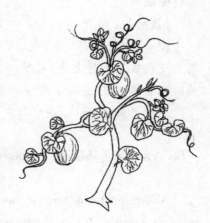

【注释】

［1］痈肿：气血受邪毒所困，壅塞不通，造成局部肿胀。

［2］金石：通过在熔岩坩锅中加热矿物质、金属和其他天然物质而制成的丹药。中国古代有人希望服用金石来保持健康和追求长寿。

## 13. Gualou ［栝蒌(瓜蒌)，snakegourd fruit，Fructus Trichosanthis］

Its seeds can promote lactation.

For abscess[1]: Boil its roots with vinegar until they are dry, mash them into powder and filter the powder. Mix the powder with vinegar, spread this out on a piece of paper and apply the paper to the abscess. The method is especially suitable for those taking Jinshi[2].

【Notes】

［1］abscess：It is a local swelling caused by stagnation of qi and blood due to evil toxin.

［2］Jinshi：It refers to the Dan medicine（elixirs）made by heating minerals, metals and other natural substances in a luted crucible. Some ancient Chinese took it in order to keep healthy and live longer.

## 14. 燕覆子(通草)　平

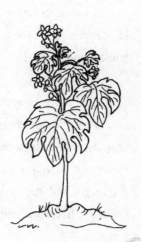

（一）右主利肠胃，令人能食。下三焦[1]，除恶气。和子食更良。江北人多不识此物，即南方人食之。

（二）又，主续五藏音声及气，使人足气力。

（三）又，取枝叶煮饮服之，治卒气奔绝。亦通十二经脉。其茎为(通)草，利关节拥塞不通之气。今北人只识通草，而不委子功。（其皮不堪食）。

（四）煮饮之，通妇人血气。浓煎三、五盏，即便通。

（五）又，除寒热不通之气，消鼠瘘[2]、金疮、踠折。

煮汁酿酒妙。

【注释】

[1] 三焦：六腑之一，是上、中、下三焦的合称，将躯干划分为三个部位：横膈以上内脏器官为上焦，包括心、肺；横膈以下至脐内脏器官为中焦，包括脾、胃、肝、胆等内脏；脐以下内脏器官为下焦，包括肾、大肠、小肠、膀胱。

[2] 鼠瘘：病症名，疾病日久而成脓溃破，进而形成窦道的淋巴结核病。

## 14. Yanfuzi [燕覆子, trifoliate akebia, Akebiae Trifoliatae Caulis] *mild*

As mentioned above, it can mainly benefit the stomach and intestine and increase appetite. It can disinhibit triple energizer[1] and dispel malign qi. It will be more effective when eating it with its seeds. It is less well known to northerners, i. e., it is more welcomed by southerners.

It can replenish insufficient healthy qi in the five zang-organs, making people stronger, more energetic and speak with resonance.

It can treat the sudden abnormal flow of qi and the depletion of the vital energy by decocting its branches and leaves and taking the decoction. It can also dredge the twelve meridians. Its stalks are called Tongcao (通草) that can disperse qi stagnation in the joints. Nowadays, northerners only use Tongcao (通草) without the knowledge of its seeds. It is not advisable to eat its skin.

Its decoction can resolve menstruation irregularities. Taking three to five bowls of the strongly made decoction can disinhibit menstrual blood.

It can also remove cold and heat, disperse qi stagnation and treat scrofula[2], injury caused by metal and fracture of the bones and sinews. It is also effective to make liquor with its decoction.

【Notes】

[1] triple energizer: One of the six fu-organs. It is the combination of upper, middle and lower energizer. According to the theory of TCM, the trunk of human body is divided into three parts. The visceral organs above the diaphragm belong to the upper energizer, including the heart and lung; the visceral organs between the diaphragm and the umbilicus belong to the middle energizer, including the spleen, stomach, liver and gallbladder; and the visceral organs below the umbilicus belong to

the lower energizer, including the kidney, large intestine, small intestine and bladder.

［2］scrofula：It is also known as mouse sores. An infective surgical disease which happens in the neck area. There are some nodes felt by pressing the skin under the neck which are connected with each other. The smaller ones are called small scrofula while the larger ones are called large scrofula. The youth and those who have already contracted tuberculosis may get this disease.

## 15. 百 合 平

主心急黄[1]，（以百合）蒸过，蜜和食之。作粉尤佳。红花者名山丹，不堪食。

【注释】

［1］心急黄：黄疸重症，病情发作暴急凶险，伴有高热、烦渴、神昏、谵语，重则嗜睡昏迷等临床表现。

## 15. Baihe〔百合, lily bulb, Bulbus Lilii〕*mild*

It can mainly treat acute jaundice[1] by steaming it and taking it with honey. It is particularly effective to grind it and take the powder. Shandan〔山丹, morningstar lily bulb, Lilii Concoloris Bulbus〕with red flowers is not edible.

【Note】

［1］acute jaundice：It is a severe case of jaundice with sudden onset, rapid deterioration and poor prognosis, accompanied by high fever, dire thirst, impairment of consciousness, delirium and even lethargy and coma.

## 16. 艾 叶

（一）干者并煎者，（主）金疮，崩中，霍乱[1]；止胎漏。春初采，为干饼子，入生姜煎服，止泻痢。三月三日，可采作煎，甚治冷。若患冷气[2]，取熟艾面裹作馄饨，可大如弹子许。

（二）（艾实）：又治百恶气，取其子，和干姜捣作末，蜜丸如梧子大，空心三十丸服，以饭三、五匙压之，日再服。其鬼神速走出，颇消一切冷气。田野之人与此方相宜也。

（三）又，产后泻血不止，取干艾叶半两炙熟，老生姜半两，浓煎汤，一服便止，妙。

【注释】

［1］霍乱：病症名，以发病突然、剧烈呕吐和腹泻为主要特征。

［2］冷气：脏腑之气与寒冷相搏所致的疾患。

## 16. Aiye［艾叶，argy wormwood leaf，Folium Artemisiae Argyi］

Both the dried and decocted Aiye［艾叶，argy wormwood leaf，Folium Artemisiae Argyi］can mainly treat the injury caused by metal, metrorrhagia and cholera[1]. It can also relieve vaginal bleeding during pregnancy. It can eliminate diarrhea and dysentery by collecting it in early spring, making dried cakes, decocting the cakes with Shengjiang［生姜，fresh ginger, Rhizoma Zingiberis Recens］and taking the decoction. It can dispel cold qi effectively by collecting and decocting it on the 3rd of the third lunar month. When suffering from cold qi[2], fry it, knead the dough with it and make wontons as big as marbles.

Aishi［艾实，mugwort fruit, Artemisiae Argyi Fructus］can also treat all kinds of malign qi. Mash it with Ganjiang［干姜，dry ginger, Rhizoma Zingiberis］into powder, make honeyed pills as big as Wutongzi［梧桐子，firmiana seed, Firmianae Semen］, take 30 pills before meals and have three to five spoons of rice to suppress their tastes, which can expel ghost qi quickly and eliminate all cold qi effectively. The method is especially suitable for those often working in the fields.

When suffering from persistent bleeding after the delivery of baby, broil half a Liang of the dried Aiye, decoct them strongly with half a Liang of Shengjiang and take the soup at a time, which will take effect instantly.

【Notes】

［1］cholera：It is a disease characterized by the sudden onset of simultaneous vomiting and diarrhea.

［2］cold qi：It is a disease caused by the mutual contention between qi of zang-fu organs and cold.

## 17．蓟菜（小蓟）

（一）小蓟根：主养气。取生根叶,捣取自然汁,服一盏,立佳。

（二）又,取菜煮食之,除风热。

（三）根主崩中。又,女子月候伤过,捣汁半升服之。

（四）叶只堪煮羹食,甚除热风气。

（五）又,金创血不止,挼叶封之即止。

（六）夏月热,烦闷不止：捣叶取汁半升,服之立瘥。

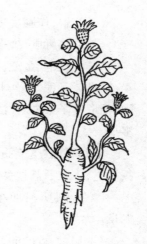

### 17. Jicai（Xiaoji）[蓟菜（小蓟）, field thistle herb, Herba Cirsii]

Its roots can mainly nourish qi. It will take effect instantly by mashing its fresh leaves and roots and taking 1 Zhan of the natural juice.

It can also eliminate wind heat by boiling it and taking the decoction.

Its roots can mainly treat metrorrhagia. It can also treat hypermenorrhea by mashing its roots and taking half a Sheng of the juice.

Its leaves can only be boiled into thick soup and are quite effective in eliminating wind heat.

It can cease bleeding caused by metal injury instantly by rubbing its leaves and applying them to the affected area.

For persistent vexation on hot summer days：Mash its leaves, take half a Sheng of the juice and you will recover instantly.

# 18．恶食（牛蒡）

（一）根，作脯食之良。

（二）热毒肿，捣根及叶封之。

（三）杖疮、金疮，取叶贴之，永不畏风。

（四）又瘫缓及丹石风毒，石热发毒。明耳目，利腰膝：则取其子末之，投酒中浸经三日，每日饮三两盏，随性多少。

（五）欲散支节筋骨烦热毒。则食前取子三七粒，熟挼吞之，十服后甚食良。

（六）细切根如小豆大，拌面作饭煮食，（消胀壅）尤良。

（七）又，皮毛间习习如虫行，煮根汁浴之。夏浴慎风。却入其子炒过，末之如茶，煎三匕[1]，通利小便。

【注释】

[1] 匕：古代的计量单位，1 匕约合今制 2～3 克。

## 18. Eshi（Niubang）[恶食（牛蒡），arctium，Arctii Fructus]

Its preserved roots are beneficial to health.

When suffering from abscess and swelling caused by heat toxin, mash its roots and leaves, and apply them to the affected area.

When suffering from the injury caused by bludgeoning or metal, apply its leaves to the affected area and you will then be resistant to wind evil for all time.

It can also treat paralysis and disperse the wind toxin caused by mineral intoxication and the heat toxin caused by Jinshi. It can improve hearing and vision and facilitate the waist and knees: Grind its seeds into powder, soak the powder in liquor for three days and take 2 or 3 Zhan of the liquor every day, but never drink too much.

It can eliminate the vexation, swelling and pain of the joints and bones. Rub twenty-one seeds repeatedly, take them for ten times successively before meals and you will recover then.

It is particularly effective in eliminating the swelling and distention in the abdomen by chopping its roots as fine as Xiaodou ［小豆, mung bean, Phaseoli Radiati Semen］, mixing them with flour, cooking and eating them.

When suffering from itching, as serious as being crawled over by bugs, decoct its roots in water and take a bath in the decoction. Be cautious of the wind when bathing in summer. It can disinhibit urination by frying its seeds, grinding them as fine as tea powder, decocting 3 Bi[1] of the powder and taking the decoction.

【Note】

［1］Bi: A unit of capacity in ancient times. 1 Bi is roughly equivalent to 2 ~ 3 grams today.

# 19. 海 藻

（一）主起男子阴气,常食之,消男子癀疾[1]。南方人多食之,传于北人。北人食之,倍生诸病,更不宜矣。

（二）瘦人,不可食之。

【注释】

［1］癀(tuí)疾:男子的睾丸肿大疼痛。

## 19. Haizao ［海藻, seaweed, Sargassum］

It can mainly enhance male sexual functions. Regular eating of it can treat scrotal swelling[1]. Southerners often eat it and then introduce it to the north. Northerners come down with a variety of diseases after eating it, which demonstrates that it is not suitable for them.

It is not suitable for lean people, either.

【Note】

［1］scrotal swelling: It is a disease characterized by swollen and painful testicles.

## 20. 昆 布

下气,久服瘦人。无此疾者,不可食。海岛之人爱食,为无好菜,只食此物。服久,病亦不生。遂传说其功于北人。北人食之,病皆生,是水土不宜尔。

### 20. Kunbu〔昆布, kelp, Thallus Laminariae〕

It can direct qi downward. Long-term taking of it can make people thin. It is not suitable for those not suffering from the disease. Islanders love and have to eat it, for there is nothing better on the island. Long-term taking of it can make people less susceptible to diseases.

Therefore, its effects have been introduced to the north. Northerners come down with a variety of diseases after eating it because of unacclimatization.

## 21. 紫 菜

下热气,多食胀人。若热气塞咽喉,煎汁饮之。此是海中之物,味犹有毒性。凡是海中菜,所以有损人矣。

### 21. Zicai〔紫菜, laver, Porphyra〕

It can clear heat qi and direct qi downward. Excessive eating of it can cause abdominal distention. Decocting it and taking the decoction can treat heat qi blocking the throat. Growing in the sea, it is still toxic in taste and property. All vegetables growing in the sea, to some extent, will do harm to health.

## 22. 船底苔

冷,无毒。治鼻洪,吐血,淋疾:以炙甘草并豉汁浓煎汤,旋呷。又,主五淋[1]:取一团鸭子大,煮服之。又,水中细苔:主天行病,心闷,捣绞汁服。
【注释】
[1] 五淋:石淋、气淋、膏淋、劳淋、血淋。

## 22. Chuanditai〔船底苔, hull bottom moss, Materia Medica Chuanditai〕

It is cold in property and is non-toxic. For nosebleed, hematemesis and stranguria：Decoct it into thick soup with Zhigancao〔炙甘草, mix-fried licorice, Glycyrrhizae Radix cum Liquido Fricta〕and fermented black soybeans and sip the soup hot. For five kinds of stranguria[1]：Choose one as large as a duck egg, decoct it and take the decoction. Tiny moss in water can mainly treat seasonal epidemic and eliminate vexation by mashing and wringing it and then taking the juice.

【Note】

〔1〕five kinds of stranguria：Urolithic stranguria, qi stranguria, chylous stranguria, overstrain stranguria and blood stranguria.

# 23. 干 苔

味咸,寒一云温。主痔,杀虫,及霍乱呕吐不止,煮汁服之。又,心腹烦闷者,冷水研如泥,饮之即止。又,发诸疮疥,下一切丹石[1],杀诸药毒。不可多食,令人痿黄,少血色。杀木蠹虫,内木孔中。但是海族之流,皆下丹石。

【注释】

〔1〕丹石:同金石,通过在熔岩坩锅中加热矿物质、金属和其他天然物质而制成的丹药。中国古代有人希望服用金石来保持健康和追求长寿。

## 23. Gantai〔干苔, enteromorpha, Enteromorphae Thallus〕

It is salty in taste and cold in property, while some people say that it is warm in property. It can mainly treat hemorrhoids, kill worms and cure cholera and persistent vomiting by boiling it and taking the decoction. It can treat vexation in the heart and abdomen by grinding it with cold water and taking the pulp. It can cause scabies, but can eliminate the toxin of Danshi[1] and remove the toxicity of various drugs as well. It is not advisable to eat more for fear of sallow complexions and looking pale. It can eliminate timbre beetles by putting it in the holes of a moth-eaten tree. Any creature growing in the sea can eliminate the toxin of Danshi.

【Note】

[1] Danshi：It is the same as Jinshi, which refers to the Dan medicine ( elixirs ) made by heating minerals, metals and other natural substances in a luted crucible. Some ancient Chinese took it in order to keep healthy and live longer.

# 24. 懷香(小茴香)

（一）（恶心）:取蘹香华、叶煮服之。

（二）国人重之,云有助阳道,用之未得其方法也。生捣茎叶汁一合,投热酒一合。服之治卒肾气[1]冲胁、如刀刺痛,喘息不得。亦甚理小肠气。

【注释】

[1] 肾气:肾精化生之气,表现为肾脏的功能活动,如生长、发育及性机能的活动。

## 24. Huaixiang (Xiaohuixiang)［懷香(小茴香)，fennel，Fructus Foeniculi］

For nausea：Decoct its flowers and leaves and take the decoction.

It is said to have the effect of enhancing male sexual functions, so it is valued by Chinese people. However, it is not well used in medical practices. Mashing its fresh stalks and leaves into 1 Ge of juice, mixing the juice with 1 Sheng of hot liquor and taking the juice can treat the sudden rising of kidney qi[1] towards the rib, the pain of which feels like being stabbed by a knife, and people will feel painful even when panting. The method is also effective in treating hernia.

【Note】

[1] kidney qi：It refers to the qi generated by kidney essence, which is manifested by functions of the kidney, such as growth, development and sexual function.

# 25. 荠 苨

丹石发动,取根食之尤良。

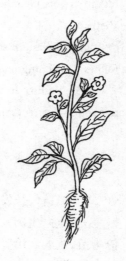

## 25. Jini〔荠苨, apricot-leaved adenophora, Adenophorae Trachelioidis Radix〕

Its roots are particularly effective in eliminating mineral intoxication.

# 26. 蒟 酱 温

散结气,治心腹中冷气。亦名土荜拨。岭南[1]荜拨尤治胃气疾[2],巴蜀[3]有之。

**【注释】**

[1] 岭南:南岭山脉以南的地区,包括广东、广西、海南以及越南北部一小部分。

[2] 胃气疾:胃的功能失调所引起的胃脘痞胀、嗳气、食欲减退等。

[3] 巴蜀:四川盆地及其附近地区,位于中国西南部,包括四川省和重庆市。

## 26. Jujiang〔蒟酱, betel pepper, Piperis Betle Fructus〕*warm*

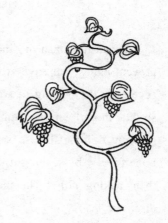

It can disperse qi bind and treat cold qi in the heart and abdomen. It is also called Tubiba（土荜拨）. Biba（荜拨） growing in Lingnan[1] is particularly effective in treating the disease of stomach qi[2], and this kind of Biba（荜拨）also grows in Bashu[3].

**【Notes】**

[1] Lingnan: It is a geographic term, referring to the area in the south of the Nanling Mountains. The

region covers Guangdong, Guangxi and Hainan as well as a small part of northern Vietnam.

［2］disease of stomach qi：It is a disease characterized by epigastric stuffiness and fullness，belching and loss of appetite，which is caused by stomach dysfunctions.

［3］Bashu：It refers to the area of Sichuan basin and its vicinity. It is located in the southwest of China，including Sichuan Province and Chongqing City.

## 27. 青蒿（草蒿） 寒

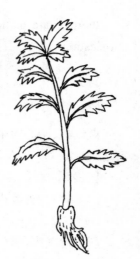

（一）益气长发，能轻身补中，不老明目，煞风毒。捣敷疮上，止血生肉。最早，春前生，色白者是。自然香醋淹为菹，益人。治骨蒸[1]，以小便渍一两宿，干，末为丸，甚去热劳[2]。

（二）又，鬼气，取子为末，酒服之方寸匕[3]，瘥。

（三）烧灰淋汁，和锻石煎，治恶疮瘢魇。

【注释】

［1］骨蒸：自感发热自骨髓蒸发而出，常见于结核病。

［2］热劳：虚劳病之呈现热象者。

［3］方寸匕：古代的计量单位，1 方寸匕约为 5 毫升。

## 27. Qinghao（Caohao）［青蒿（草蒿），sweet wormwood herb，Herba Artemisiae Annuae］ *cold*

It can replenish qi，increase hair growth，relax the body，tonify the middle，prevent aging，improve vision and disperse wind toxin. It can cease bleeding and accelerate the healing of sores by mashing and applying it to the affected area. It sprouts in early spring with white tender buds. It can nourish the human body by pickling it into Chinese sauerkraut with aromatic vinegar. It can treat steaming bone fever[1] by soaking it in urine for one or two days，drying and grinding it，and then making pills. The method is also effective in treating pyretic consumptive disease[2].

The powder of its seeds, taken with 1 Fangcunbi (square-cun-spoon)[3] of liquor, works well on treating ghost qi.

It can treat severe sores, scars and melanotic nevus by burning it into ash, filtering the ash with water and making decoction with lime.

**【Notes】**

[1] steaming bone fever: It is a disease where patients feel fever deep in the body emanating from the bone or marrow seemingly, which is commonly found in subcutaneous node.

[2] pyretic consumptive disease: It is a kind of consumptive disease where heat is represented.

[3] Fangcunbi (square-cun-spoon): A unit of capacity in ancient times. 1 Fangcunbi is about 5 milliliter.

## 28. 菌 子 寒

（一）发五脏风壅经脉，动痔病，令人昏昏多睡，背膊、四肢无力。

（二）又，菌子有数般，槐树上生者良。野田中者，恐有毒，杀人。

（三）又，多发冷气，令腹中微微痛。

### 28. Junzi〔菌子, meadow mushroom, Agaricus Campestris〕*cold*

It can cause wind evil in the five zang-organs blocking the channels and cause hemorrhoids. It can make people feel drowsy and have weak shoulders, backs and limbs.

It has several types, and the better one is on pagoda trees. Be cautious of the one growing in the wild, for it may be toxic and even fatal.

It can also stir cold qi frequently, resulting in dull pain in the abdomen.

## 29. 牵牛子

多食稍冷，和山茱萸服之，去水病[1]。

**【注释】**

[1] 水病：即水肿病，是以肌肤浮肿为主要表现的疾病的统称。

## 29. Qianniuzi〔牵牛子, pharbitis seed, Semen Pharbitidis〕

Excessive eating of it can damage yang qi and cause aversion to cold. Taking it with Shanzhuyu〔山茱萸, asiatic cornelian cherry fruit, Fructus Corni〕can treat edema[1].

〔**Note**〕

〔1〕edema：It is a disease characterized by subcutaneous fluid retention.

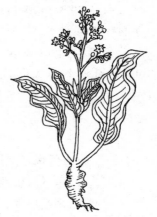

## 30. 羊　蹄

主痒，不宜多食。

## 30. Yangti〔羊蹄, root of Japanese dock, Radix Rumicis〕

It can mainly relieve itching, but is not suitable to eat more.

## 31. 菰菜、菱首[1]

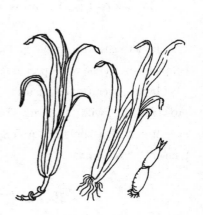

（一）菰菜：利五脏邪气，酒皶面赤，白癞[2]疬疡[3]，目赤等效。然滑中，不可多食。热毒风气[4]，卒心痛，可盐、醋煮食之。

（二）若丹石热发，和鲫鱼煮作羹，食之三两顿，即便瘥耳。

（三）菱首：寒。主心胸中浮热风，食之发冷气，滋人齿，伤阳道，令下焦冷滑[5]，不食甚好。

【注释】

〔1〕菰菜、菱首：菰菜感染黑粉菌后无法抽穗，其茎部逐渐膨大形成菱首。

〔2〕白癞：麻风病的一种类型，初起皮色逐渐变白、四肢麻木、肢节发热、手足无力，或声音嘶哑、两眼视物不清。

[3] 疬疡:又名"疬疡风",症见面颊颈项忽生斑驳,点点相连而圆,似癣。

[4] 风气:风邪侵身,包括外风和内风。外风是自然风邪侵入人体所致,内风则是脏腑功能失调所致,尤其是肝功能失调和气血运动失调所致。

[5] 下焦冷滑:下焦的脏腑虚寒而出现腹泻、白带清稀、滑精等症状。

## 31. Gucai, Jiaoshou[1] [菰菜、荻首, infested ear of wild rice, Zizaniae Spica Infestata]

It can dispel evil qi in the five zang-organs and treat rosacea, red face, tuberculoid leprosy[2], pyogenic infection of skin[3], redness of the eyes, etc. However, it is not suitable to eat more, for it will cause spleen-stomach weakness of the middle energizer. It can disperse heat toxin and wind qi[4] and treat sudden heart pain by boiling it with salt and vinegar and taking the decoction.

When suffffering from mineral intoxication, boil it into the thick soup with Jiyu [鲫鱼, crucian carp, Carassii Aurati Caro], take the soup for two or three times and you will recover then.

It is cold in property. It can treat floating heat wind in the heart and chest. Eating it can cause cold qi, damage the teeth, hamper male sexual functions and cause the lower energizer slippery cold[5]. It is better not to eat it.

【Notes】

[1] Gucai, Jiaoshou: Gucai cannot ear after being infected with smut fugus, and its stems grow gradually into Jiaoshou.

[2] tuberculoid leprosy: It is a type of leprosy characterized by gradual whitening of the skin, numbness of the limbs, fever of the limbs and joints, weakness of the hands and feet, hoarseness of the voice and unclear vision.

[3] pyogenic infection of skin: There are blotches on the skin of the face and neck which connect into circles and are similar to tinea.

[4] wind qi: It refers to the wind evil invading the body. It includes the external wind qi and the internal wind qi. The external wind qi is caused by the natural wind evil invading the body, and the internal wind qi is caused by the dysfunction of zang-fu organs, especially by the liver dysfunction and the movement disturbance of qi and blood.

［5］ lower energizer slippery cold：It refers to diarrhea, clear-thin vaginal discharge, spontaneous seminal emission and other symptoms caused by deficiency cold of the lower energizer.

# 32. 萹竹（萹蓄）

（一）蚘虫心痛，面青，口中沫出，临死：取叶十斤[1]，细切；以水三石三斗，煮如饧，去滓。通寒温，空心服一升，虫即下。至重者再服，仍通宿勿食，来日平明服之。

（二）患痔：常取萹竹叶煮汁澄清。常用以作饭。

（三）又，患热黄、五痔[2]：捣汁顿服一升，重者再服。

（四）丹石发，冲眼目肿痛：取根一握，洗。捣以少水，绞取汁服之。若热肿处，捣根茎敷之。

【注释】

［1］斤：计量单位，1 斤相当于 500 克。

［2］五痔：病症名，肛门痔五种类型之合称。《备急千金要方》卷二十三曰："夫五痔者，一曰牡痔，二曰牝痔，三曰脉痔，四曰肠痔，五曰血痔。"

## 32. Bianzhu（Bianxu）［萹竹（萹蓄），common knotgrass herb，Herba Polygoni Avicularis］

When suffering from heart pain caused by roundworms, green-blue complexion, frothing at the mouth and impending death, chop 10 Jin[1] of its leaves finely, boil them with 3 Dan and 3 Dou of water into the decoction as sticky as the syrup and filter the decoction. Take 1 Sheng of the decoction before meals when the temperature is appropriate, and the roundworms will be eliminated along with the stool. Take that decoction again, but do not eat anything all night and wait to take it again early the next day when seriously affected.

When suffering from hemorrhoids, usually decoct its leaves, filter the decoction and cook rice with it.

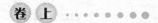

For damp-heat jaundice and five kinds of hemorrhoids[2]: Mash it and take 1 Sheng of the juice at a time. Take it again when seriously affected.

For the swelling and pain of eyes caused by mineral intoxication: Wash a full handful of its roots, mash them with a little water, twist them and take the juice. Mash its stalks and roots and apply them to the affected area if there is a local fever and swelling.

【Notes】

[1] Jin: A unit of capacity in ancient times. 1 Jin is equivalent to 500 grams.

[2] five kinds of hemorrhoids: A collective term of hemorrhoids of five kinds. In Volume 23 of *Bei Ji Qian Jin Yao Fang* [《备急千金要方》, *Essential Recipes for Emergent Use Worth a Thousand Gold*] says that there are five kinds of hemorrhoids: male hemorrhoid, female hemorrhoid, pulse hemorrhoid, intestine hemorrhoid and blood hemorrhoid.

## 33. 甘　蕉

主黄疸。子:生食大寒。主渴,润肺,发冷病[1]。蒸熟暴之令口开,春取人食之。性寒,通血脉,填骨髓。

【注释】

[1] 冷病:虚寒病,指由于阳气虚弱而导致的一系列"寒象"及功能活动低下。

### 33. Ganjiao [甘蕉, banana, Musae Paradisiacae Fructus]

It can mainly treat jaundice. Its raw fruit is severely cold in property. It can mainly relieve thirst, moisten the lung and cause deficiency cold[1]. Steam it, expose it to the sun until it cracks, mash it to get kernels and take them. Its kernels are cold in property and can promote blood circulation and enrich marrow.

【Note】

[1] cold disease: It is also called deficiency-cold syndrome. It refers to a series of cold manifestations and hypofunction.

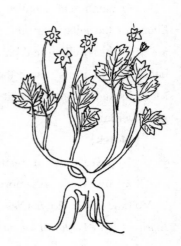

## 34. 蛇 莓

（一）主胸、胃热气,有蛇残不得食。

（二）主孩子口噤[1],以汁灌口中,死亦再活。

【注释】

[1] 口噤:病症名,指牙关紧闭、口不能张开
的症状。

### 34. Shemei［蛇莓, snake strawberry,

### Duchesneae Herba］

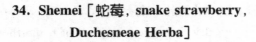

It can mainly eliminate heat qi in the chest and stomach. When bitten and left with the venom of the snake, it will not be edible.

It can mainly treat the clenched jaw[1] of children by feeding them with its juice, and even the dying one can be saved with it.

【Note】

[1] clenched jaw: It is a symptom characterized by lockjaw and inability to open the mouth.

## 35. 苦 芙 微寒

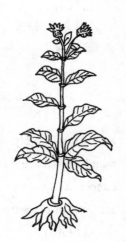

生食治漆疮[1]。五月五日采,暴干作灰,敷面目、通
身漆疮。不堪多食尔。

【注释】

[1] 漆疮:病症名,皮肤感受漆毒后出现以红斑、脱
屑、瘙痒等为主要特征的疾病。

### 35. Ku'ao〔苦芺，Chinese thistle，Cirsii Chinensis Herba〕*slightly cold*

Raw Ku'ao〔苦芺，Chinese thistle，Cirsii Chinensis Herba〕can treat lacquer sore[1]. Pick it on the 5th of the fifth lunar month, dry it and burn it into ash. The ash is then applied to the sore of the face, eyes or the whole body. It is not suitable to eat more.

【Note】

[1] lacquer sore: It is a disease characterized by erythema, desquamation and itching due to lacquer toxin.

## 36. 槐 实

（一）主邪气，产难，绝伤。

（二）春初嫩叶亦可食，主瘾疹[1]，牙齿诸风疼。

【注释】

[1] 瘾疹：隐疹，病症名，是以皮肤出现风团、瘙痒时隐时现为主要特征的过敏性皮肤病。

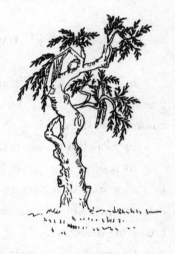

### 36. Huaishi〔槐实，fruit of pagodatree，
### Fructus Sophorae〕

It can mainly treat diseases caused by evil qi, difficult delivery of babies and fracture of the bones and sinews.

Its tender buds collected in early spring are also edible and can mainly treat urticaria[1] and toothache caused by severe wind evil.

【Note】

[1] urtucaria: It is a disease characterized by an allergic disorder of the skin, marked by red or pale wheals and intermittent itching.

# 37. 枸 杞 寒

（一）无毒。叶及子：并坚筋能老，除风，补益筋骨，能益人，去虚劳。

（二）根：主去骨热，消渴[1]。

（三）叶和羊肉作羹，尤善益人。代茶法煮汁饮之，益阳事。

（四）能去眼中风痒赤膜，捣叶汁点之良。

（五）又，取洗去泥，和面拌作饮，煮熟吞之，去肾气[2]尤良。又益精气。

## 【注释】

[1] 消渴：病症名，类似于西药中的糖尿病，泛指以多饮、多食、多尿、形体消瘦或尿有甜味为特征的疾病。

[2] 肾气：肾气不固，症见尿频遗尿、男子遗精滑泄、女子月经淋沥不止等。

## 37. Gouqi [枸杞，fruit of barbary wolfberry，Fructus Lycii] *cold*

It is non-toxic. Its leaves and fruit can strengthen the sinews and bones, prevent aging, dispel wind evil, nourish the human body and eliminate consumptive disease.

Its roots can mainly treat steaming bone fever and consumptive thirst[1].

Its leaves are particularly effective in nourishing the human body when made into thick soup with Yangrou [羊肉，goral flesh，Naemorhedi Goral Caro]. It can enhance male sexual functions by decocting its leaves, just like brewing tea, and taking the decoction.

It can effectively treat both itchy eyes and redness of the eyes due to wind toxin by mashing its leaves and applying the juice to the eyes.

To treat kidney qi insecurity[2] and replenish essential qi, wash out the mud on its roots, chop them finely, mix them with flour, make soup and take it.

## 【Notes】

[1] consumptive thirst：A disease similar to diabetes in Western medicine. It is characterized by polydipsia, polyphagia, polyuria, emaciation or sweet urine.

[2] kidney qi insecurity：It is a syndrome marked by frequent urination, dribbling of urine after voiding, nocturnal emission or premature ejaculation in men and continuous dribbling of menstruation.

## 38. 榆 荚 平

（一）右疗小儿痫疾[1]，（小便不利）。

（二）又方，患石淋[2]、茎又暴赤肿者：榆皮三两，熟捣，和三年米醋滓封茎上。日六七遍易。

（三）又方，治女人石痈[3]、妒乳肿[4]。

（四）案经：宜服丹石人。取叶煮食，时服一顿亦好。高昌[5]人多捣白皮为末，和菹菜食之甚美。消食，利关节。

（五）又，其子可作酱，食之甚香。然稍辛辣，能助肺气。杀诸虫，下（气[6]，令人能食。又）心腹间恶气，内消之。陈滓者久服尤良。

（六）又，涂诸疮癣妙。

（七）又，卒冷气心痛，食之瘥。

【注释】

[1] 痫疾：癫痫，症见突然倒地、口吐白沫、手足痉挛，发作后即可恢复正常。

[2] 石淋：病症名，指小便涩痛，尿出砂石。

[3] 石痈：病症名，痈肿坚硬如石。

[4] 妒乳肿：乳痈，病症名，指痈肿之发于乳房者。

[5] 高昌：一处古老的已被废弃的绿洲城市遗址，位于新疆吐鲁番东南30千米处。

[6] 气：胃气，指中医理论中的胃肠消化功能。

## 38. Yujia [榆荚, dwarf elm fruit, Ulmi Pumilae Fructus] *mild*

As mentioned above, it can treat epilepsy[1] and dysuria.

For urolithic stranguria[2] and sudden swelling of penis: Mash 3 Liang of Yupi [榆皮, bark of Chinese elm, Cortex Ulmi Parvifoliae], mix them with dregs of rice vinegar stored for three years and apply them to the penis for six or seven times a day.

It can also treat oncoma[3] and acute mastitis[4] of women.

The following is supplemented by Zhang Ding: It is suitable for those taking

Danshi. It can also be effective to boil its leaves irregularly and take the decoction. Those living in Gaochang[5] often mash Yubaipi 〔榆白皮, bark of Chinese elm, Cortex Ulmi Parvifoliae〕 into powder and eat the powder with Chinese sauerkraut, which tastes delicious and can stimulate digestion of food and soothe the joints.

Its seeds can be made into sauce, which tastes delicious, but a bit spicy. The sauce can disinhibit lung qi, kill worms, direct stomach qi[6] downward and increase appetite. The sauce can also allow malign qi in the heart and abdomen to be absorbed internally. It will be more effective when eating the sauce with dregs of years.

The sauce is also effective in treating sore and tinea.

The sauce can treat the sudden heart pain caused by cold qi instantly.

**〔Notes〕**

〔1〕 epilepsy：It is a disease characterized by falling down suddenly, frothing at the mouth, spasm of hands and feet and returning to normal shortly after the onset.

〔2〕 urolithic stranguria：It is a disease characterized by painful and difficult urination due to the passage of urinary calculi.

〔3〕 oncoma：It is a disease characterized by the swelling as hard as a rock.

〔4〕 acute mastitis：It is a disease characterized by the swelling on the breast.

〔5〕 Gaochang：It is the site of a ruined, ancient oasis city located 30 km southeast of Tulufan in Xinjiang, China.

〔6〕 stomach qi：The gastrointestinal digestive function according to the theory of TCM.

# 39. 酸 枣 平

主寒热结气,安五藏,疗不能眠。

## 39. Suanzao 〔酸枣, spiny jujube, Ziziphi Spinosi〕 *mild*

It can mainly disperse qi stagnation caused by cold and heat, pacify the five zang-organs and cure insomnia.

## 40. 木 耳 寒

无毒。利五藏,宣肠胃气拥、毒气,不可多食。惟益服丹石人。热发,和葱豉作羹。

### 40. Mu'er〔木耳, golden tremella, Tremella Mesenterica〕*cold*

It is non-toxic. It can harmonize the five zang-organs, disperse qi stagnation in the intestine and stomach and remove toxic qi. It is not advisable to eat more. It is only beneficial to those taking Danshi and can eliminate mineral intoxication by eating the thick soup made with scallions and fermented black soybeans.

## 41. 桑

(一)桑椹:性微寒。食之补五藏,耳目聪明,利关节,和经脉,通血气,益精神。

(二)桑根白皮:煮汁饮,利五藏。又入散用,下一切风气水气[1]。

(三)桑叶:炙,煎饮之止渴,一如茶法。

(四)桑皮:煮汁可染褐色,久不落。柴:烧灰淋汁入炼五金家用。

【注释】

[1] 水气:古代的水肿病。

### 41. Sang〔桑, mulberry, Morus alba L.〕

Sangshen〔桑椹, mulberry fruit, Fructus Mori〕is slightly cold in property. Eating it can tonify the five zang-organs, improve hearing and vision, soothe the joints, harmonize the channels, promote the circulation of blood and nourish essence and spirit.

Sanggen Baipi〔桑根白皮, bark of white mulberry, Cortex Mori〕: Boil it, take the decoction to harmonize the five zang-organs then. It can also dispel all wind qi and water qi[1] by grinding it and taking the powder.

Sangye〔桑叶, mulberry leaf, Folium Mori〕: Broil it, decoct it with water, take the decoction to relieve thirst then. The method of making and using it is the same as that of tea.

Sangpi〔桑皮, mulberry bark, Mori Cortex〕: Its boiled decoction can be used as the brown dye, and the dyed objects do not fade even after a long time. Firewood: Burn it into ash and filter the ash with water. The method is always used by alchemists.

【Note】

［1］water qi: An ancient disease which is also called edema.

# 42. 竹

（一）淡竹上,甘竹次。主咳逆[1],消渴,痰饮[2],喉痹[3],鬼疰[4]恶气。杀小虫,除烦热。

（二）苦竹叶:主口疮,目热,喑哑。

（三）苦竹茹:主下热壅。

（四）苦竹根:细锉一斤,水五升,煮取汁一升,分三服。大下心肺五藏热毒气。

（五）笋:寒。主逆气,除烦热,又动气,能发冷症,不可多食。越有芦及箭笋,新者稍可食,陈者不可食。其淡竹及中母笋虽美,然发背闷脚气。

（六）苦笋不发痰。

（七）竹笋不可共鲫鱼食之,使笋不消成症病,不能行步。

（八）慈竹:夏月逢雨,滴汁著地,生蓐似鹿角,色白。取洗之,和姜酱食之,主一切赤白痢[5]。极验。

（九）慈竹沥:疗热风,和食饮服之良。

（十）淡竹沥:大寒。主中风大热,烦闷劳复。

（十一）淡竹茹:主噎膈[6],鼻衄。

（十二）竹实:箪通神明,轻身益气。

（十三）箪、淡、苦、甘外,余皆不堪,不宜人。

【注释】

［1］咳逆:病症名,指咳嗽见气上逆的疾患。

［2］痰饮:病症名,指体内水液输布运化失常,停积于某些部位。

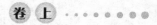

［3］喉痹：病症名，主要表现为咽部红肿疼痛，或干燥、异物感，或咽痒不适、吞咽不利。

［4］鬼疰(zhù)：突发心腹刺痛，重则闷绝倒地，并能传染他人的病症。

［5］赤白痢：病症名，下痢黏胨脓血，赤白相杂。

［6］噎膈：饮食吞咽不利，梗塞难下，或食物入胃即吐。

## 42. Zhu［竹，bamboo，Bambusoideae］

Danzhu［淡竹，lophatherum herb，Herba Lophatheri］is the best and is followed by Ganzhu［甘竹，bambusa schreb.，Materia Medica Ganzhu］. It can mainly treat cough with dyspnea[1], consumptive thirst, phlegm-fluid retention[2], pharyngitis[3], demonic infixation[4] and malign qi. It can also kill small worms and eliminate vexation.

Kuzhuye［苦竹叶，bitter bamboo leaf，Pleioblasti Folium］can mainly treat aphtha, redness of the eyes and loss of voice.

Kuzhuru［苦竹筎，bitter bamboo shavings，Pleioblasti Caulis in Taenis］can mainly dispel the binding of heat toxin.

Kuzhugen［苦竹根，bitter bamboo root，Pleioblasti Rhizoma］: File 1 Jin of Kuzhugen, mix them with 5 Sheng of water into 1 Sheng of juice and take the juice for three times. The method is quite effective in dispersing heat toxin and evil qi.

Sun［笋，bamboo shoot，Bambusae Surculus］is cold in property. It can mainly treat the counterflow of qi and eliminate vexation. It is also easy to stir qi and cause the binding of cold qi. Therefore, it is not advisable to eat more. Yue (now Zhejiang Province in China) has Lusun［芦笋，phragmites shoot，Phragmititis Surculus］and Jiansun［箭笋，usawa cane shoot，Pseudosasae Usawai Surculus］. They are edible when fresh, but will not be so if stored for a long time. Danzhusun［淡竹笋，bamboo shoot，Bambusae Surculus］and Zhongmusun are delicious, but will cause the stuffy pain of the back and weak foot.

Kusun［苦笋，bitter bamboo shoot，Pleioblasti Caulis］will not cause diseases caused by phlegm.

Zhusun［竹笋，bamboo shoot，Bambusae Surculus］cannot be eaten together with Jiyu〔鲫鱼, crucian carp, Carassii Aurati Caro〕. Eating the two together will cause indigestion, binding in the abdomen and inability to walk.

Cizhu〔慈竹, bambusa emeiensis, Materia Medica Cizhu〕: Its juice drops on the ground and then sprouts when raining in summer, and its white buds look like antlers. Its buds can effectively treat red and white dysentery[5] by washing first and taking them together with Shengjiang〔生姜, rhizome of common ginger, Rhizoma Zingiberis Recens〕and sauce.

Cizhuli〔慈竹沥, sap of bambusa emeiensis, Materia Medica Cizhuli〕can expel heat wind and will be more effective when taking it together with food and rice soup.

Danzhuli〔淡竹沥, bamboo sap, Bambusae Succus〕is severely cold in property. It can mainly treat wind stroke, severe heat and recurring vexation caused by overstrain.

Danzhuru〔淡竹筎, bamboo shavings, Bumbusae Caulis in Taenia〕can mainly treat dysphagia[6] and epistaxis.

Zhushi〔竹实, bamboo fruit, Bumbusae Fructus〕can invigorate spirit and mentality, relax the body and replenish qi.

Bamboos are inedible, except Jinzhu〔箽竹, top-grade bamboo, Materia Medica Jinzhu〕, Danzhu〔淡竹, lophatherum herb, Herba Lophatheri〕, Kuzhu〔苦竹, bitter bamboo leaf, Pleioblasti Folium〕and Ganzhu〔甘竹, bambusa schreb., Materia Medica Ganzhu〕.

【Notes】

〔1〕cough with dyspnea: It is a syndrome characterized by cough with counterflow of qi in the airways.

〔2〕phlegm-fluid retention: It is a disease which refers to the abnormal flow of phlegm and fluid in the human body and the consequent retention of phlegm and fluid in any part of the body.

〔3〕pharyngitis: It is a disease characterized by the redness, swelling and pain of the throat, the dry throat with a sensation of having something there, or the itching the of throat with impediment to swallowing.

〔4〕demonic infixation: It is a syndrome characterized by sudden pain in the heart and abdomen, and unconsciousness and falling down in severe cases, which can infect others.

[5] red and white dysentery: A disease with symptoms of fever, abdominal pain and stool with mucus, pus and blood.

[6] dysphagia: It is a disease characterized by difficulty in swallowing caused by narrowing or obstruction of the esophagus, or instant vomiting.

## 43. 吴茱萸 温

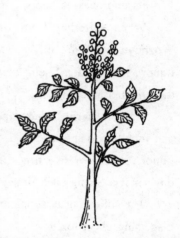

（一）右主治心痛，下气，除咳逆，去藏中冷。能温脾气[1]消食。

（二）又方，生树皮：上牙疼痛痒等，立止。

（三）又，（患风[2]瘙痒痛者），取茱萸一升，清酒五升，二味和煮，取半升去滓，以汁微暖洗。

（四）如中风贼风[3]，口偏不能语者，取茱萸一升，美清酒四升，和煮四五沸，冷服之半升。日二服，得小汗为瘥。

（五）案经：杀鬼毒尤良。

（六）又方：夫人冲冷风欲行房，阴缩不怒者，可取二七粒，（嚼）之良久，咽下津液。并用唾涂玉茎头即怒。

（七）又，闭目者名榝子，不宜食。

（八）又方，食鱼骨在腹中，痛，煮汁一盏，服之即止。

（九）又，鱼骨刺在肉中不出，及蛇骨者，（捣吴茱萸）以封其上，骨即烂出。

（十）又，奔豚气[4]冲心，兼脚气上者[5]，可和生姜汁饮之，甚良。

（十一）微温。主痢，止泻，厚肠胃。肥健人不宜多食。

【注释】

[1] 脾气：脾的功能及其赖以产生的精微物质或动力。

[2] 风：风疹，是由风疹病毒引起的急性传染病，多见于幼儿。

[3] 贼风：四季的气候异常所引发的风邪。

[4] 奔豚气：病症名，指有气从少腹上冲胸及咽喉，发作欲死，腹痛，发作后复如常人。

[5] 脚气上者：脚气冲心，是脚气病的危症，主要表现为心悸气喘、面唇青紫、神志恍惚和恶心呕吐。

## 43. Wuzhuyu〔吴茱萸, medicinalevodia fruit, Fructus Evodiae〕*warm*

As mentioned above, it can mainly treat heart pain, direct qi downward, eliminate cough with dyspnea and dispel cold qi in the zang-fu organs. It can warm spleen qi[1] and stimulate the digestion of food.

Its unprocessed barks can also cease toothache and tooth itching instantly.

When suffering from rubella[2] with pain and itching, boil 1 Sheng of Wuzhuyu〔吴茱萸, medicinalevodia fruit, Fructus Evodiae〕with 5 Sheng of clear liquor, filter half a Sheng of the decoction, heat the decoction slightly and wash the affected area with it.

When suffering from wind stroke, thief wind[3], mouth drooping on one side and inability to speak, boil 1 Sheng of Wuzhuyu with 4 Sheng of superlative clear liquor for four or five times, cool the decoction, take the decoction two times a day, half a Sheng each time, and you will recover after sweating a little.

The following is supplemented by Zhang Ding: It is particularly effective in dispersing ghost toxin.

When suffering from inability to get an erection in sexual intercourse after being blown by a cold wind, chew fourteen Wuzhuyu for a period of time, swallow the spittle and smear it on the glans penis, which will help them get an erection instantly.

The one whose crust does not crack is called Dangzi (櫃子), which is not edible.

When suffering from pain caused by fish bones stuck in the abdomen, take 1 Zhan of its decoction and you will recover instantly.

When suffering from inability to pull fish or snake bones out of the human flesh, mash and apply it to the affected area, and then the bones can be softened and removed.

When suffering from running piglet[4] affecting the heart and disease of weak foot affecting the heart[5], take its juice together with the juice of Shengjiang〔生姜, rhizome of common ginger, Rhizoma Zingiberis Recens〕, which can be quite effective.

It is slightly warm in property. It can mainly treat dysentery, cease diarrhea and invigorate the intestine and stomach. It is not suitable for obese and healthy people to eat more.

【Notes】

[1] spleen qi: The function of the spleen as well as the nutrient substance and the driving force from which the function comes.

[2] rubella: It is an acute infectious skin disease caused by rubella virus. It often occurs to children and is characterized by red rashes all over the body.

[3] thief wind: It refers to the wind evil caused by the abnormal weather in the four seasons.

[4] running piglet: It is a disease characterized by qi ascending from the lower abdomen to the chest and throat, near-death experiences and abdominal pain. Patients will return to normal after the attack.

[5] disease of weak foot affecting the heart: It is a severe case of weak foot, which is characterized by palpitation, asthma, a pale appearance, blue lips, trance, nausea and vomiting.

## 44. 食茱萸 温

（一）主心腹冷气痛，中恶[1]，除咳逆，去藏腑冷，能温中[2]，甚良。

（二）又，齿痛，酒煎含之。

（三）又，杀鬼毒。中贼风，口偏不语者，取子一升，美豉三升，以好酒五升，和煮四五沸，冷服半升，日三四服，得汗便瘥。

（四）又，皮肉痒痛。酒二升，水五升，茱萸子半升，煎取三升，去滓微暖洗之立止。

（五）又，鱼骨在腹中刺痛，煎汁一盏服之，其骨软出。

（六）又，脚气冲心，和生姜煎汁饮之。

（七）又，鱼骨刺入肉不出者，捣封之。其骨自烂而出。

（八）又，闭目者名榝子，不堪食。

【注释】

[1] 中恶：因感受秽毒或不正之气而突然厥逆，不省人事。

[2] 温中：以温补药物来治疗脾胃阳虚证的方法。

## 44. Shizhuyu〔食茱萸, ailanthus zanthoxylum fruit, Zanthoxyli Ailanthoidis Fructus〕 *warm*

It can mainly treat the pain caused by cold qi in the heart and abdomen, cure the attack of noxious factor[1], eliminate cough with dyspnea, dispel cold qi in the zang-fu organs and warm the middle[2].

It can also treat toothache by decocting it with liquor and taking the decoction.

It can disperse ghost toxin. When suffering from thief wind, mouth drooping on one side and inability to speak, boil 1 Sheng of its seeds with 3 Sheng of superlative fermented black soybeans and 5 Sheng of superlative rice liquor for four or five times, cool the decoction, take the decoction three or four times a day, half a Sheng each time, and you will recover after sweating a little.

When suffering the pain and itching of skin, decoct half a Sheng of its seeds with 2 Sheng of rice liquor and 5 Sheng of water into 3 Sheng of decoction, filter the decoction, heat the decoction slightly, wash the affected area with decoction and recover instantly.

When suffering from the pain caused by fish bones in the abdomen, take 1 Zhan of its decoction, and the fish bones will then be softened and removed.

When suffering from the disease of weak foot affecting the heart, decoct it with Shengjiang〔生姜, rhizome of common ginger, Rhizoma Zingiberis Recens〕 and take the decoction.

When suffering from inability to pull fish or snake bones out of the human flesh, mash and apply it to the affected area, and then the bones can be softened and removed.

The one whose crust does not crack is called Dangzi (樣子), which is not edible.

**〔Notes〕**

〔1〕attack of noxious factor: It is a disease which is manifested as reversal cold of limbs and unconsciousness caused by dirt, poison and unhealthy qi.

〔2〕warm the middle: It is a therapeutic method to treat the yang deficiency of the spleen and stomach with warm-tonifying medication.

## 45. 槟 榔

多食发热,南人生食。闽中名橄榄子。所来北者,煮熟,熏干将来。

### 45. Binlang〔槟榔, areca seed, Semen Arecae〕

Excessive eating of it can cause heat toxin. Southerners eat raw Binlang〔槟榔, areca seed, Semen Arecae〕. It is called Ganlanzi（橄榄子）in Minzhong（now Fujian Province in China）. It is cooked, smoked and dried in the south before transporting to the north.

## 46. 栀 子

（一）主喑哑,紫癜风[1],黄疸,积热心躁。

（二）又方,治下鲜血,栀子人烧成灰,水和一钱匕[2]服之,量其大小多少服之。

**【注释】**

[1] 紫癜风:病症名,皮肤上出现紫红色的扁平皮疹、瘙痒,常累及口腔。

[2] 钱匕:古代量取药末的器具。用汉代的五铢钱币量取药末至不散落为一钱匕;用五铢钱匕量取药末至半边者为半钱匕。钱五匕,是指药末盖满五铢钱边的"五"字至不落为度。一钱匕大概 2 克多;半钱匕大概 1 克多;钱五匕大概 0.6 克。

### 46. Zhizi〔栀子, cape jasmine fruit, Fructus Gardeniae〕

It can mainly treat loss of voice, purple patch wind[1], jaundice and vexation caused by accumulation of heat.

It can also treat bloody stool by burning its seeds into ash and mixing 1 Qianbi[2] of the ash with water. The amount to be taken will vary with the age and amount of stool blood.

**【Notes】**

[1] purple patch wind: It is a disease characterized by flat burgundy rashes and

itching, often involving the mouth.

［2］Qianbi：An ancient coin. Its surface can be used for measuring the amount of medicinal powder. 1 Qianbi is about 2 grams, and 1 Banqianbi（half a Qianbi）is about 1 gram. 1 Qianwubi is about 0.6 gram.

## 47. 芜 荑 平

（一）右主治五内邪气，散皮肤支节间风气。能化食，去三虫[1]，逐寸白，散腹中冷气。

（二）又，患热疮[2]，为末和猪脂涂，瘥。

（三）又方，和白沙蜜治湿癣[3]。

（四）又方，和马酪治干癣[4]，和沙牛酪疗一切疮。

（五）案经：作酱食之，甚香美。其功尤胜于榆人，唯陈久者更良。可少吃，多食发热、心痛，为其味辛之故。秋天食之（尤）宜人。长吃治五种痔病。（诸病不生）。

（六）又，杀肠恶虫。

【注释】

［1］三虫：蛔虫、蛲虫、赤虫（姜片虫）三种常见的肠寄生虫。

［2］热疮：病症名，指发热或高热过程中出现在皮肤黏膜交界处的急性疱疹性皮肤病。

［3］湿癣：病症名，风湿热邪侵入肌肤而引发的皮肤潮红、糜烂、瘙痒不止等症状。

［4］干癣：病症名，一种慢性的顽固性皮肤病。

### 47. Wuyi ［芜荑，great elm seed，Semen Ulmus Macrocarpa］ *mild*

As mentioned above, it can mainly treat diseases in the five zang-organs caused by evil qi and disperse the retention of wind qi in the skin and joints. It can digest food, expel three worms[1], eliminate tapeworms and disperse cold qi in the abdomen.

When suffering from heat sore[2], grind it, mix its powder with Zhuyou ［猪油，pork lard，Suis Adeps］, apply the powder to the sore and recover then.

It can also treat damp lichen[3] by mixing it with light white substances left by the long-stored sugar.

It can also treat dry lichen[4] by mixing it with the horse cheese. It can also treat all sores by mixing it with the cow milk cheese.

The following is supplemented by Zhang Ding: It tastes quite delicious and has far more effects than Yurenjiang〔榆仁酱, dwarf elm fruit jam, Ulmi Pumilae Fructus Praeparatio〕when made into sauce. It is better to keep it longer. It is advisable to eat less. Excessive eating of it can cause heat toxin and heart pain, because it is pungent in taste. Eating it in autumn can better nourish the human body. Eating it for a long time can treat five kinds of hemorrhoids and prevent diseases.

It can also expel evil worms in the intestines.

【Notes】

〔1〕 three worms：Intestinal parasites including roundworm, pinworm and redworm.

〔2〕 heat sore：It is an acute herpetic dermatosis referring to the growing of vesicles on the junction of the skin and mucosa complicated with fever or hyperthermia.

〔3〕 damp lichen：It is a disease caused by wind dampness and wind evil, which will result in symptoms such as redness, anabrosis and the itching of the skin.

〔4〕 dry lichen：It is a chronic refractory skin disease.

# 48. 茗(茶)

（一）茗叶：利大肠，去热解痰。煮取汁，用煮粥良。

（二）又，茶主下气，除好睡，消宿食，当日成者良。蒸、捣经宿。用陈故者，即动风发气。市人有用槐、柳初生嫩芽叶杂之。

## 48. Ming（Cha）〔茗(茶)，tea，Theae Folium〕

It can disinhibit the large intestine, clear heat and dispel phlegm. It is good to make porridge with the tea water.

It can also direct qi downward, reduce fatigue and stimulate the digestion of retained food. Brewing and drinking tea on that very day can be more effective. Steaming and mashing the tea, then leaving it for a whole night, or using the old tea will cause diseases due to wind evil. Some dealers blend the tender buds of pagoda trees or willows with it on the market.

## 49. 蜀椒[1]·秦椒[2] 温

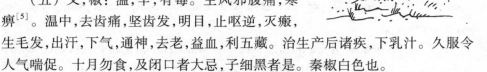

（一）粒大者,主上气咳嗽,久风湿痹[3]。

（二）又,患齿痛,醋煎含之。

（三）又,伤损成疮中风,以面裹作馄饨,灰中炮之,使熟断开口,封其疮上,冷,易热者,三五度易之。亦治伤损成弓风[4]。

（四）又去久患口疮,去闭口者,以水洗之,以面拌煮作粥,空心吞之三、五匙,（以）饭压之。（重者可）再服,（以）瘥（为度）。

（五）又,椒:温,辛,有毒。主风邪腹痛,寒痹[5]。温中,去齿痛,坚齿发,明目,止呕逆,灭瘢,生毛发,出汗,下气,通神,去老,益血,利五藏。治生产后诸疾,下乳汁。久服令人气喘促。十月勿食,及闭口者大忌,子细黑者是。秦椒白色也。

（六）除客热[6],不可久食,钝人性灵。

【注释】

[1] 蜀椒:属芸香科植物,出武都及巴郡,又名“巴椒”。

[2] 秦椒:因出自秦地(甘肃天水一带),故称“秦椒”。

[3] 风湿痹:病名。由于风寒湿热等外邪入侵,闭阻经络关节,导致气血运行不畅,全身关节呈游走性红、肿、疼痛。

[4] 弓风:病名。风毒侵入人体,导致全身肌肉持久性强直痉挛,使身体仰曲如弓。

[5] 寒痹:病名,又名“痛痹”“骨痹”。寒邪偏重,气血凝滞不通,导致肢体关节疼痛,遇寒加重,得热痛减或缓解。

[6] 客热:外来的热邪,又指虚热或假热。

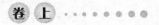
### 49. Shujiao[1] · Qinjiao[2] [蜀椒 · 秦椒, fruit of Sichuan red pepper · Qin pepper, Fructus Capsici Frutescentis Sichuan · Qin Xanthoxylum Piperitum] *warm*

The large-grained pepper can be used to treat panting and cough with qi ascent and chronic wind-dampness impediment[3].

The decoction of pepper with vinegar can be used to treat toothache.

To treat wound infection with wind toxin, it is advisable to batter the pepper with flour to make it into wonton and bake the wonton in warm ash. Break the well-done wonton and apply it on the sore. Replace the cooler wonton with hotter one and repeat that for three to five times. This method can also be used to treat tetanus[4].

It can also be used to treat long-suffered aphtha. When using, weed out the uncracked peppers. Wash the cracked ones with water, mix them with flour to make into gruel. Take three to five spoons of the gruel on an empty stomach and then take meal to ease its side effect. Seriously ill patients can keep taking it before healing.

Pepper, also known as Qin pepper, is pungent in taste, and warm and toxic in property. It is mainly used to treat wind evil complicated by abdominal pain and cold impediment[5]. Its clinical functions include warming the middle energizer, relieving toothache, strengthening teeth and hair, improving vision, ceasing retching counterflow, eliminating scar, engendering hair, inducing sweating, descending qi, invigorating spirit, dispelling blood stasis, tonifying the blood and benefiting the five zang-organs. It can also be used to treat various post-natal diseases and promote lactation. Long-term taking of it will cause hasty panting. Do not take it in the tenth lunar month, and it is a taboo to take the uncracked peppers. The fruit of Sichuan red pepper has thin and black seeds, and Qin pepper has white seeds.

It can relieve visiting heat[6], but it is not suitable to have a long-time taking, or it will cause spirit torpor.

**【Notes】**

［1］Shujiao：The genus of the Rutaceae. It originally existed in Wudu and Bajun, so it is also known as Bajiao.

［2］Qinjiao：It originally existed in the area of Qin（the area surrounding today's Tianshui of Gansu Province）, so it is called Qin pepper.

［3］wind-dampness impediment：A disease caused by invasion of external evil which will obstruct channels and network vessels as well as the joints, inhibit qi and blood, and thus cause wandering reddening, swelling and pain of joints across the whole body.

［4］tetanus：A disease caused by the invasion of wind toxin which will cause lasting and generalized muscular rigidity and spasm and thus make the back arched.

［5］cold impediment：A disease also known as painful impediment or bone impediment. Severe cold evil obstructs qi and blood, causing pain in the joints of limbs, which is exacerbated by exposure to cold and relieved by exposure to heat.

［6］visiting heat：Extraneous heat evil, also known as vacuity heat or false heat.

# 50. 蔓　椒[1]

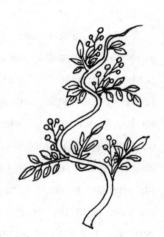

主贼风挛急[2]。

**【注释】**

［1］蔓椒：属芸香科植物,味苦,性温,主要用于跌打损伤、风湿痹病。

［2］挛急:病症名,指肌肉紧张或抽动。

## 50. Manjiao[1]［蔓椒, root of shiny bramble, Radix Shinyleaf Pricklyash］

It is mainly used to treat thief wind and hypertonicity[2].

**【Notes】**

［1］Manjiao：The genus of the Rutaceae. Bitter in taste and warm in property, it is mainly used to treat the injury caused by knocks and falls, and wind-dampness impediment.

[2] hypertonicity：A disease that refers to muscle tension or twitches.

## 51. 椿 温

（一）动风,熏十二经脉、五藏六腑。多食令人神不清,血气微。

（二）又,女子血崩及产后血不止,月信来多,可取东引细根一大握洗之,以水一大升煮,分再服便断。亦止赤带下[1]。

（三）又,椿俗名猪椿。疗小儿疳痢[2],可多煮汁后灌之。

（四）又,取白皮一握,仓粳米五十粒,葱白一握,甘草三寸炙,豉两合。以水一升,煮取半升,顿服之。小儿以意服之。枝叶与皮功用皆同。

【注释】

[1] 赤带下:病症名。在非行经期,阴道内流出赤色或赤白相间的黏液。

[2] 小儿疳痢:病症名,小儿疳疾合并痢疾。多因饮食不洁、寒温失调所致。病状主要有面黄肌瘦、精神不振、皮肤干燥、头发发黄、腹泻,并伴有脓血、粘液、腹胀、腹痛等。

### 51. Chun［椿，toon，Ailanthusaltissima（Mill.）Swingle］ *warm*

It can stir wind, and fume the twelve channels, the five zang-organs and six fu-organs. Excessive taking will make the spirit-mind unclear and cause the debilitation of blood and qi.

For flooding, persistent bleeding after delivery and heavy menstrual blood, it is advisable to wash a full handful of thin eastward roots and decoct them with 1 Sheng of water. Taking the decoction twice can staunch bleeding. This method is also effective in checking red vaginal discharge[1].

It is also known as Zhuchun（猪椿）. Taking its decoction is effective in treating infantile Gan dysentery[2].

Take a handful of the root bark of it, fifty grains of rice from granary, a handful of scallion white, 3 Cun of broiledlicorice, and 2 Ge of fermented soybean. Decoct them with 1 Sheng of water to half a Sheng of decoction, and take them one time. Children can take whatever amount suitable to them. The effect of its branches and leaves is the same to that of the root bark.

【Notes】

［1］red vaginal discharge：A syndrome that refers to the red or red-white discharge from vagina during non-menstrual period.

［2］infantile Gan dysentery：A disease referring to the combination of infantile Gan disease and dysentery. It is mainly caused by taking unclear food and disharmony of cold and warmth. The symptoms include yellow face and emaciated flesh, depression, dry skin, hair yellowing, diarrhea complicated with pus and blood, mucus and abdominal distention and pain, etc.

## 52. 樗[1]

主疳痢,杀蛔虫。又名臭椿。若和猪肉、热面频食,则中满[2],盖壅经脉也。

【注释】

［1］樗(chū):俗称"臭椿",味苦,性温,有小毒,主洗疮疥、风疽。

［2］中满:病症名,指因饮食停滞所致的脘腹胀满。

## 52. Chu[1][樗, ailanthus, Ailanthus Altissima]

It is mainly used to treat Gan dysentery and kill roundworm. It is also known as Chouchun（臭椿）. Frequent taking of it with pork and fresh wheat flour will cause center fullness[2] as it obstructs the meridians.

【Notes】

［1］Chu：Also known as Chouchun. Bitter in taste, warm and slightly toxic in property, it is mainly used to relieve scabies and wind flat-abscess.

［2］center fullness：A disease referring to distention in stomach duct and abdomen caused by stagnation of food.

## 53. 郁李人[1]（仁）

（一）气结者,酒服人四十九粒,更泻,尤良。

（二）又,破癖气[2],能下四肢水。

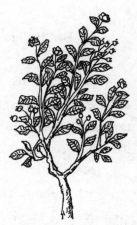

【注释】

〔1〕郁李人:即郁李仁,郁李属蔷薇科植物,郁李人(仁)就是其种仁。味苦、甘,性平,有润肺滑肠、下气利水的功效。

〔2〕癖气:病症名。饮食不节,寒痰凝聚,气血瘀阻导致痞块生于两肋,时痛时止。

## 53. Yuliren[1]〔郁李人(仁), Chinese dwarf cherry seed, Semen Pruni〕

The patients suffering from qi stagnation can take 49 grains of it with liquor. Better effects can be achieved through several more times of diarrhea.

It can be used to eliminate the fixed lump[2] and the water swelling of four limbs.

【Notes】

〔1〕Yuliren: The seed of the dwarf flowering cherry which is the genus of the Rosaceae. Pungent and bitter in taste and mild in property, it is effective in moistening the lung and lubricating the intestines, precipitating qi and disinhibiting water.

〔2〕fixed lump: A disease caused by irregular diet, congealing and stagnation of cold phlegm and obstruction of qi and blood. The fixed lump is thus engendered at both sides of the chest with irregular pain.

## 54. 胡 椒[1]

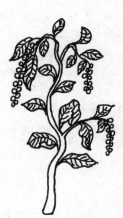

治五藏风冷,冷气心腹痛,吐清水,酒服之佳。亦宜汤服。若冷气,吞三七枚。

【注释】

〔1〕胡椒:属胡椒科,味辛,性热,有温中散寒、下气、消痰的功效。

## 54. Hujiao[1]〔胡椒, pepper fruit, Fructus Piperis Nigri〕

It is used to treat the wind cold of the five zang-organs, the pain in heart and abdomen caused by cold qi, and the vomiting of clear water. Taking it with liquor can achieve good effects. It is also appropriate for decoction. To eliminate cold qi, the patient can take 21 grains of it.

【Note】

[1] Hujiao：The genus of the Piperaceae. Pungent in taste and hot in property, it is effective in warming the center and dissipating cold, precipitating qi and dispersing phlegm.

## 55. 橡 实[1]

主止痢,不宜多食。

【注释】

[1] 橡实:壳斗科植物麻栎的果实,味苦,性微温,有收敛固涩、止血、解毒之功效。

## 55. Xiangshi[1]〔橡实, acorn, Quercus Acutissimae Fructus〕

It is mainly used to check dysentery, and it is inappropriate to take it excessively.

【Note】

[1] Xiangshi：The fruit of Mali〔麻栎, german oak, Quercus Acutissima Carruth〕which is Fagaceae plant. Bitter in taste and slightly warm in property, it is effective in astringing astriction, stanching bleeding and resolving toxin.

## 56. 鼠 李[1] 微寒

(一)主腹胀满。其根有毒,煮浓汁含之治䘌齿。并疳虫[2]蚀人脊骨者,可煮浓汁灌之食。

（二）其肉：主胀满谷胀[3]，和面作饼子，空心食之，少时当泻。

（三）其煮根汁，亦空心服一盏，治脊骨疳[4]。

【注释】

[1] 鼠李：属鼠李目植物，味苦，微寒，有清热利湿、消积杀虫之效。

[2] 疳虫：古人认为小儿疳疾皆由乳哺不调、寒温失节而使腹内生虫所致。

[3] 谷胀：病症名，又称"食胀"，因食物不消化导致胸腹胀满。

[4] 脊骨疳：病症名。由于久患疳疾，消耗骨肉导致极度消瘦，脊骨突出似锯。

## 56. Shuli[1][鼠李，davurian buckthorn fruit，Fructus Rhamni Davuricae] *slightly cold*

It is mainly used to treat abdominal fullness and distention. Holding its thick decoction of root, which is toxic, in mouth can treat tooth decay. To treat Gan worms[2] eating into spines, drink its thick decoction of root.

Its flesh is mainly used to treat fullness and grain distention[3]. Mix it with flour to make pancakes and take them on an empty stomach. It doesn't take long time to drain the accumulated food.

Taking 1 Zhan of its decoction of root can treat the Gan of spines[4].

【Notes】

[1] Shuli：The genus of the Rhamnales. Bitter in taste and slightly cold in property, it is effective in clearing heat and disinhibiting dampness, dispersing accumulations and killing worms, etc.

[2] Gan worms：The ancients believed that the Gan disease in children was caused by worms in the abdomen and the worms was caused by irregular breast feeding and abnormal heat and cold.

[3] grain distention：A disease also known as food distention. It refers to fullness and distention in chest and abdomen caused by non-transformation of food.

[4] Gan of spines：A disease caused by the chronic Gan disease which exhausts blood and flesh and thus makes the spines protruding like a saw.

# 57. 枳　椇[1]

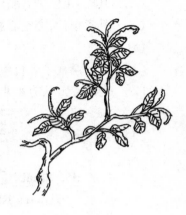

多食发蛔虫。昔有南人修舍用此,误有一片落在酒瓮中,其酒化为水味。

【注释】

[1] 枳椇:属鼠李科枳椇属植物,以树皮和种子入药,味甘,性平。枳椇树皮有活血、舒筋解毒之效。枳椇子有清热利尿、止渴除烦、解酒毒之效。

## 57. Zhiju[1]［枳椇, honey tree, Hoveniaacerba Lindl.］

Taking it excessively will cause the roundworm. Someone from the South once used it to build a house while one piece accidentally fell into the liquor jar, making the liquor taste like water.

【Note】

[1] Zhiju：The genus of the Rhamnaceae Hovenia. Its bark and seeds are used as medicine. It is pungent in taste and mild in property. Its bark is effective in activating blood, soothing the sinews and resolving toxin. Its seeds are effective in clearing heat and disinhibiting urine, relieving thirst and eliminating vexation, and resolving liquor toxin.

# 58. 棐（榧）子[1] 平

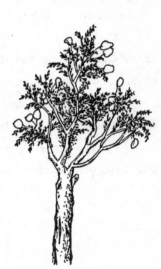

(一) 右主治五种痔,去三虫,杀鬼毒,恶疰[2]。

(二) 又,患寸白虫人,日食七颗,经七日满,其虫尽消作水即瘥。

(三) 按经:多食三升、二升佳,不发病。令人消食,助筋骨,安荣卫[3],补中益气,明目轻身。

【注释】

[1] 棐（榧）子:属红豆杉科植物,味甘,性平,

有杀虫消积、润肺止咳、润燥通便之效。

［２］恶疰：病症名。身体虚弱，被恶毒之气所伤，流移至心腹，导致持续疼痛。

［３］荣卫：营卫。荣，同"营"，指营气和卫气。荣指血的循环，卫指气的周流，荣卫二气散布全身，对人体起着滋养和保卫的作用。

## 58. Feizi[1][榧（榧）子, torreya, Torreyae Semen] *mild*

It is mainly used to treat five kinds of hemorrhoids, to eliminate three worms, and to kill ghost toxin and toxin infixation[2].

People suffering from inch white worms can take seven grains per day for seven consecutive days before all the worms will be transformed into water.

The following is supplemented by Zhang Ding：Taking 2 or 3 Sheng more can achieve better effects without causing other diseases. It can disperse food accumulations, strengthen sinews and bones, harmonize Rongwei[3], tonify the middle, replenish qi, improve vision and relax the body.

【Notes】

［１］Feizi：The genus of the Taxaceae. Pungent in taste and mild in property, it is effective in killing worms and dispersing accumulation, lubricating the lung and suppressing cough, moistening dryness and freeing the stool.

［２］toxin infixation：A disease occurs when the toxic qi invades the weak body, spreads to the heart region and abdomen, and causes persistent pain.

［３］Rongwei：Rong refers to the blood circulation and Wei refers to the qi movement. Rong qi（nutrient-qi）moves in the vessels, so it is yin and Wei qi（defensive-qi）runs out of the vessels, so it is yang. Rong and Wei function together and endlessly to nurture and defend the body.

## 59. 藕 寒

（一）右主补中焦，养神，益气力，除百病。久服轻身耐寒，不饥延年。

（二）生食则主治霍乱后虚渴、烦闷、不能食。长服生肌肉，令人心喜悦。

（三）案经：神仙家[1]重之，功不可说。其子能益气，即神仙之食，不可具说。

（四）凡产后诸忌，生冷物不食。唯藕不同生类也。为能散血之故。但美即而已，可以代粮。

（五）（又），蒸食甚补益（五藏，实）下焦，令肠胃肥厚，益气力。与蜜食相宜，令腹中不生诸虫。

（六）（亦可休粮[2]）。仙家有贮石莲子[3]及干藕经千年者，食之不饥，轻身能飞，至妙。世人何可得之。凡男子食，须蒸熟服之，生吃损血。

【注释】

[1] 神仙家：中国古代为追求"长生不死"而通过吐纳呼吸、服食丹药、草药等方式进行"修炼"的术士，始于春秋战国时期。

[2] 休粮：古人常用的一种养生方式，又称"辟谷"。在不吃五谷的同时，通过摄入坚果、草药等对身体机能进行调节。

[3] 石莲子：属睡莲科，味甘，性涩，有清湿热、开胃进食、清心宁神、涩精止泻等功效。

### 59. Ou〔藕，lotus root，Nelumbinis Rhizoma〕*cold*

It is mainly used to tonify the middle energizer, nourish spirit, replenish qi and energy, and eliminate all diseases. Long-term taking of it can relax the body, tolerate cold and hunger, and prolong life.

Eating its raw fruit can eliminate cholera-incurring vacuity and thirst, vexation and oppression, and inability to eat. Long-term taking of it can engender muscles and maintain good mood.

The following is supplemented by Zhang Ding: In ancient times, the alchemists[1] attached great importance to it and kept its functions secrete. Its seeds can boost qi, and therefore they were made food for the alchemists, but its functions could not let the public know in details.

All kinds of postpartum taboos of food, especially raw and cold ones, are prohibited. It is the only exception as it can dissipate blood and replace grains, but do not take much.

Taking the steamed one can tonify the five zang-organs and the lower energizer, thicken the stomach and intestines, and replenish qi and energy. It is appropriate to take it with honey, which can repel all worms in the abdomen.

(It can also be used for inedia[2].) It is said that alchemists who ate Shilianzi[3] [石莲子, lotus fruit, Nelumbinis Fructus] and dry Ou [藕, lotus root, Nelumbinis Rhizoma] that had been stored for thousands of years had no feeling of hunger and were full of vigor as if flying. That is really amazing and unapproachable for common people. Male must take the steamed one, as taking the raw one can cause blood loss.

【Notes】

[1] alchemist: (in the original text), it refers to the warlocks who, starting from the period of the Spring and Autumn, and the Warring States, cultivated themselves in ways of regulating breathing, taking exilirs and herbs, etc. to pursue immortality.

[2] inedia: A health preservation method of eating nuts and herbal medicines instead of grains. The purpose of it is to dispel turbid qi and regulate the functions of body. It is regarded by alchemists as a method of pursuing immortality in ancient times.

[3] Shilianzi: The genus of the Nymphaeaceae. Sweet in taste and astringent in property, it is effective in clearing damp-heat, increasing the appetite, clearing the heart and tranquilizing the mind, astringing essence and checking diarrhea, etc.

# 60. 莲 子[1] 寒

（一）右主治五藏不足，伤中[2]气绝，利益十二经脉、廿五络血气。生吃（微）动气，蒸熟为上。

（二）又方，（熟）去心，曝干为末，著蜡及蜜，等分为丸服。（日服三十丸），令（人）不饥。学仙人最为胜。

（三）若雁腹中者，空腹服之七枚，身轻，能登高涉远。采其雁（食）之，或粪于野田中，经年犹生。

（四）又，或于山岩石下息、粪中者，不逢阴雨，数年不坏。

（五）又，诸飞鸟及猿猴，藏之于石室之内，其猨、鸟死后，经数百年者，取得之服，永世不老也。

（六）其子房及叶皆破血<sup>[3]</sup>。

（七）又，根停久者，即有紫色。叶亦有褐色，多采食之，令人能变黑如瑿。

**【注释】**

［1］莲子：属睡莲科植物，味甘、涩，性平，有补脾止泻、止带、益肾涩精、养心安神之效。

［2］伤中：病症名，指内脏或膈的损伤，也指中焦脾胃功能的损伤，此处指内脏之气受损。

［3］破血：中医活血法之一，指用比较峻烈的药物祛瘀滞、散症结。

## 60. Lianzi[1] [莲子, lotus seed, Nelumbinis Semen] *cold*

It is mainly used to supplement insufficiency of the five zang-organs, treat damage to the middle[2] and failure of zang qi, and boost the blood and qi of the twelve channels and the twenty-five network vessels. Taking it raw will slightly stir qi, so it is better to steam it before taking it.

Another formula: Remove its plumule after steaming it, sun-dry it, grind it to powder, make pills with the equal part of wax and honey. Taking 30 pills per day will make people tolerate hunger. This formula is most favored by those who cultivate immortality.

On an empty stomach, take seven grains of it taken from the stomach of wild geese, which can relax the body to climb and hike far. Those eaten by wild geese and then defected to the field can still sprout even years later.

Those taken from the droppings of wild geese which take a rest under the mountain rocks are not rotten even years later if not exposed to rain.

Some birds, apes and monkeys used to hide it in stone caverns. Finding out and taking it even several hundred years after those animals died enable people to live a long life.

Both its ovaries and leaves are effective in breaking blood[3].

The lotus roots will turn purple overtime, and the lotus leaves will turn brown. Eating purple roots and brown leaves more than enough will make the skin dark and glossy like amber.

**【Notes】**

［1］Lianzi: The genus of the Nymphaeaceae. Sweet in taste, astringent and mild in property, it is effective in tonifying the spleen and checking diarrhea, checking vaginal discharge, supplementing the kidney and astringing essence, nourishing the heart and quieting the spirit.

［2］damage to the middle: A deficiency disease caused by the injury of internal organs.

［3］breaking blood: A blood-activating method in traditional Chinese medicine to use strong medicine to eliminate blood stasis and disperse concretions and binds.

# 61. 橘 温

（一）（穰）：止泄痢。食之，下食，开胸膈痰实结气。下气不如皮也。穰不可多食，止气。性虽温，甚能止渴。

（二）皮：主胸中瘕热逆气。

（三）又，干皮一斤，捣为末，蜜为丸。每食前酒下三十丸，治下焦冷气。

（四）又，取陈皮[1]一斤，和杏仁[2]五两，去皮尖[3]熬，加少蜜为丸。每日食前饮下三十丸，下腹藏间虚冷气。脚气冲心[4]，心下结硬，悉主之。

【注释】

［1］陈皮：橘的干燥成熟果皮，味苦、辛，性温，有理气健脾、燥湿化痰之效。

［2］杏仁：杏的种仁，味苦，微温，有小毒，有止咳平喘、润肠通便之效。

［3］去皮尖：杏仁等种仁类中药的炮制方法，即去掉外层种皮和胚芽，旨在更好地煎出药材有效成分。

［4］脚气冲心：病症名。脚气迁移失治、邪毒上攻心胸导致心悸气喘、面唇青紫、神志恍惚、恶心呕吐、腿脚微软等。

# 61. Ju ［橘, tangerine, Citrus Reticulata］ *warm*

Its segments can be used to treat diarrhea. Taking it can promote digestion and dissipate phlegm-heat stagnation and qi stagnation in the chest and diaphragm. It is less effective than its peel in promoting qi to descend. Do not take too much of it as it will cause qi stagnation. In spite of its warm property, it is very effective in relieving thirst.

Its peel is mainly used to treat accumulation of heat and counterflow of qi in the chest.

Grind 1 Jin of dry peel into powder, and make it into pills with honey. Taking 30 pills with liquor before meal can treat the cold qi of the lower energizer.

Take 1 Jin of Chenpi[1] 〔陈皮, dried tangerine peel, Pericarpium Citri Reticulatae〕 and 5 Liang of seed-coat-and-germ-removed[2] Xingren[3] 〔杏仁, bitter apricot seed, Semen Armeniacae Amarum〕. After decocting them together, add in a small amount of honey to make into pills. Taking 30 pills per day before meal can precipitate the vacuity cold qi of the lower abdomen organs. It is also effective in treating weak foot affecting the heart[4] and hard bind below the chest.

【Notes】

［1］Chenpi: The dry and ripened peel of Ju 〔橘, tangerine, Citrus Reticulata〕. Bitter and pungent in taste and warm in property, it is effective in rectifying qi and fortifying the spleen, and drying dampness and transforming phlegm.

［2］removing seed coat and germ: A processing method for seed-type medicinal herb (such as Xingren) which refers to removing the seed coat and germ, with the purpose to extract the active constituents in decoction.

［3］Xingren: The seed of apricot. Bitter in taste, slightly warm and toxic in property, it is effective in suppressing cough and calming panting, moistening the intestines and freeing the stool.

［4］weak foot affecting the heart: A syndrome caused by lack of proper treatment of leg qi. The toxin evil moves upward to the chest, causing symptoms such as palpitation and panting, green-blue or purple cheeks and lips, abstraction, nausea and vomiting, limp legs and feet, etc.

# 62. 柚[1]

味酸,不能食。可以起盘。

【注释】

［1］柚:属芸香科植物,味甘、酸,性寒,有消食、化痰、醒酒之功效。

## 62. You[1]［柚，pomelo，Citrus Maxima（Burm）Merr.］

Sour in taste, it is inedible but can be put in a tray for sacrifice.

【Note】

［1］You: The genus of the Rutaceae. Sweet and sour in taste and cold in property, it is effective in promoting digestion, resolving phlegm and dispelling the effects of liquor.

## 63. 橙[1] 温

（一）去恶心，胃风[2]：取其皮和盐贮之。

（二）又，瓢：去恶气。和盐蜜细细食之。

【注释】

［1］橙：属芸香科植物，味酸性凉，有和胃降逆、宽胸开结、消瘿、解鱼蟹毒等功效。

［2］胃风：病名，指风邪中于胃，导致腹泻、多汗、恶风等症状，或因胃中积热生风，以呕吐为主证。

## 63. Cheng[1]［橙，orange，Citrus Sinensis］ *warm*

To treat nausea and stomach wind[2], pickle its peel with salt and take it.

Its flesh can expel the malign qi. Mix it with salt and honey, and take it slowly.

【Notes】

［1］Cheng: The genus of the Rutaceae. Sour in taste and cool in property, it is effective in harmonizing the stomach and downbearing counterflow, loosening the chest and dissipating binds, dispersing goiter, resolving the toxin of fish and crabs, etc.

［2］stomach wind: A disease caused by wind evil invading the stomach. The symptoms include diarrhea, sweating, aversion to wind, etc. Or it is caused by accumulation of heat in the stomach which engenders wind and the chief symptom is vomiting.

# 64. 干 枣[1] 温

（一）主补津液[2]，养脾气，强志。三年陈者核中仁：主恶气、卒疰忤[3]。

（二）又，疗耳聋、鼻塞，不闻音声、香臭者：取大枣十五枚，去皮核；蓖麻子[4]三百颗，去皮。二味和捣，绵裹塞耳鼻。日一度易，三十余日闻声及香臭。先治耳，后治鼻，不可并塞之。

（三）又方，巴豆[5]十粒，去壳生用。松脂[6]同捣，绵裹塞耳。

（四）又云，洗心腹邪气，和百药毒。通九窍，补不足气。

（五）生者食之过多，令人腹胀。蒸煮食之，补肠胃，肥中益气。第一青州[7]，次蒲州[8]者好。诸处不堪入药。

（六）小儿患秋痢[9]，与虫枣食，良。

（七）枣和桂心[10]、白瓜仁、松树皮为丸，久服香身，并衣亦香。

**【注释】**

［1］干枣：干燥成熟的枣，属鼠李科植物，味甘，性平，有补益脾胃、滋养阴血、养心安神、缓和药性之效。

［2］津液：机体一切正常水液的总称，包括各脏腑形体官窍的内在液体及其正常的分泌物，是构成人体和维持生命活动的基本物质之一。

［3］疰忤：病名，犹中恶，指有传染性且病程长的慢性病。

［4］蓖麻子：属大戟科植物，味甘辛，性平，有消肿拔毒、泻下通滞之效。

［5］巴豆：味辛，性温，主治伤寒、温疟、寒热病，能破除症瘕，能解除坚硬的聚积和结滞，能治疗留饮所致癖证、腹部积水肿胀，能荡涤五脏六腑，能开通闭塞，能通利大小便，能去掉恶肉，能祛除鬼毒蛊注等各种邪物。

［6］松脂：马尾松、油松等植物木材中的油树脂，味苦，性温，主治恶性痈疮、头部溃疡、白秃，能消解风气所致之疥疮瘙痒，能安静五脏，能消除热邪所致之病。

［7］青州：古地名，"九州"之一，指泰山以东至渤海的一片区域。

［8］蒲州：古地名，今山西省永济县西南一带。

［9］秋痢：病症名。小儿脾胃嫩弱，内为乳食所伤，秋燥侵入，导致里急后重，腹痛便脓。

［10］桂心：肉桂树皮里层，味辛甘，性热，有引血化汗化脓、益精明目、消瘀生肌等功效。

## 64. Ganzao[1] [干枣，dry jujube，Fructus Ziziphi Jujubae] *warm*

It is mainly used to tonify body fluids[2], nourish spleen qi and improve memory. The seeds in three-year-old jujube pits can treat malign qi and chronic malignity stroke[3].

To treat deafness, nasal congestion and inability to hear or smell, pound 15 grains of peeled and pit-removed jujubes and 300 grains of peeled Bimazi[4] [蓖麻子，castor bean，Ricini Semen] together to a paste, wrap them with Mian [绵，silk floss，Bombycis Lana] and put them in the nostrils or ears, replace them every day. Then, hearing and smelling can be restored over 30 days later. Do not put the paste in the nostrils and ears at the same time: ears first, and then noses.

Another formula: Take 10 grains of raw Badou[5] [巴豆，croton，Fructus Crotonis], peel them, pound them with Songzhi[6] [松脂，colophony，Colophonium], wrap the paste with Mian [绵，silk floss，Bombycis Lana] and put it in ears.

It is also effective in dispelling evil qi in the heart and abdomen, and harmonizing various toxins of medicinals. It can disinhibit the nine orifices and supplement insufficient qi.

Eating too many fresh jujubes will cause abdominal distention. Eating the steamed jujubes can tonify the stomach and intestines, strengthen the middle and replenish qi. The jujubes produced from Qingzhou[7] are the best, and those produced in Puzhou[8] are next only to them. The jujubes that grow in other places cannot be used as medicine.

To treat autumn dysentery[9] in children, take worm-bitten jujubes, which is quite effective.

Long-term taking of the pills made by Jujubes, Guixin[10] [桂心，shaved cinnamon bark，Cinnamomi Cortex Rasus], pumpkin seeds and pine bark can make the body, and even the clothes, smell fragrant.

**[Notes]**

[1] Ganzao: Dry and ripened jujubes, the genus of the Rhamnaceae. Sweet in taste and mild in property, it is effective in tonifying the spleen and stomach,

nourishing yin blood, nourishing the heart, quieting the spirit and moderating the property of medicinals.

[2] body fluids: A collective term referring to all the normal fluids in human body. They include the inner fluids of the organs, body parts and orifices and their secretions, constituting one of the basic substances for the human body and its vital movement.

[3] malignity stroke: A disease, which is also called visiting hostility, caused by the invasion of foul toxicity and unright qi which make people have cold limbs and become unconscious.

[4] Bimazi: The genus of the Euphorbiaceae. Sweet and pungent in taste and mild in property, it is effective in dispersing swelling and drawing toxin, draining precipitation and freeing stagnation.

[5] Badou: Pungent in taste and warm in property, it is mainly used to treat cold damage, warm malaria and cold-heat disease, to break conglomeration, stagnated aggregation and hard accumulation, retention of fluid with hypochondriac lump and enlarged abdomen due to retention of water, to scour the five zang-organs and six fu-organs, to unobstruct block and closure, to promote urination and defecation, to remove necrotic muscles and to eliminate vicious toxin like ghost and accumulation of worms and evil factors.

[6] Songzhi: The oleoresin of trees like masson pines and Chinese pines. Bitter in taste and warm in property, it is mainly used to treat gangrene, severe sore, head ulcer, white head tinea and scabies and itching caused by wind qi, to harmonize the five zang-organs and to eliminate the diseases caused by heat evil.

[7] Qingzhou: The name of an ancient place, one of the nine states in ancient China. It covers the area ranging from Mount Tai in the west to the Bohai Sea in the east.

[8] Puzhou: The name of a place in ancient China. It refers to the area surrounding the southwest of today's Yongji County of Shanxi Province.

[9] autumn dysentery: The name of a syndrome. Since children's spleen and stomach are delicate, interior damage due to food and milk and autumn dryness cause abdominal urgency and rectal heaviness, abdominal pain and stool containing pus.

[10] Guixin: The inner bark of the cassia barktree. Pungent and sweet in taste

and hot in property, it is effective in conducting blood, eliminating sweating and pus, boosting essence and brightening eyes, dispersing stasis and engendering flesh.

# 65. 软　枣[1] 平

多食动风[2],令人病冷气,发咳嗽。

【注释】

[1] 软枣:味甘、涩,性凉,有止咳除痰、清热解毒、健胃之效。

[2] 动风:病症名,指因风阳、火热、阴血亏虚等导致肢体抽搐、眩晕、震颤等症状。

## 65. Ruanzao[1] [软枣, dateplum persimmon, Diospyroslotus L.] *mild*

Taking it excessively will cause wind stirring[2], diseases due to cold qi and coughing.

【Notes】

[1] Ruanzao: Sweet in taste, astringent and cool in property, it is effective in suppressing cough and eliminating phlegm, clearing heat and resolving toxin, and fortifying the stomach.

[2] wind stirring: A disease caused by wind yang, fire heat and yin-blood deficiency, with the symptoms of convulsion of limbs, dizziness, tremor, etc.

# 66. 蒲桃(葡萄)　平

(一)右益藏气,强志,疗肠间宿水,调中。

(二)按经:不问土地,但取藤,收之酿酒,皆得美好。

(三)其子不宜多食,令人心卒烦闷,犹如火燎。亦发黄病[1]。凡热疾后不可食之。眼暗、骨热,久成麻疖病[2]。

(四)又方,其根可煮取浓汁饮之,(止)呕哕及霍乱后恶心。

(五)又方,女人有娠,往往子上冲心[3]。细细饮之即止。其子便下,胎安好。

【注释】

[1] 黄病:病症名。瘀热宿食相搏导致身体面目皆变黄色。

［2］麻疖病:病名,即疖病,指以疖多发、反复发作、缠绵不愈为主要表现的疾病。

［3］子上冲心:病症名,又称"子悬"或"胎上逼心"。因肝郁、脾虚等使气血不和、胎气上逆,从而导致妊娠胸胁胀满、喘急、烦躁不安等。

## 66. Putao ［蒲桃(葡萄)，fruit of European grape，Fructus Vitis Viniferae］ *mild*

It can replenish zang qi, improve memory, treat intestinal water accumulation and regulate the middle.

The following is supplemented by Zhang Ding: The grapevine, wherever it is produced, can be used to make good liquor.

Excessive taking is inappropriate as it will cause acute burning-like vexation and oppression in the heart as well as xanthosis[1]. People suffering from heat disease should not take it as it will cause dim vision and bone fever which will progress to furunculosis[2] over time.

Another formula: Taking the thick decoction of its root can treat retching as well as nausea due to cholera.

Another formula: Pregnant women often have upsurge of the fetus into the heart[3]. Taking the decoction of its roots slowly can lower and quiet the fetus and thus treat the upsurge.

【Notes】

［1］xanthosis: A disease referring to yellowing of the whole body caused by contention of stagnated heat and retained food.

［2］furunculosis: A disease manifested with frequently-occurring, recurrent and continous furuncle that is hard to be recovered.

［3］upsurge of the fetus into the heart: A disease also known as chest distention during pregnancy. Causes like liver depression and spleen deficiency induce disharmony of qi and blood and fetal qi ascending counterflow, and thus result in distention and fullness in the chest and rib-side, rapid panting and dysphoria during pregnancy.

# 67. 栗 子

（一）生食治腰脚。蒸炒食之，令气拥，患风水气[1]不宜食。

（二）又，树皮：主瘅疮毒[2]。

（三）谨按：宜日中曝干，食即下气，补益。不尔犹有木气，不补益。就中吴[3]栗大，无味，不如北栗也。其上薄皮，研，和蜜涂面，展皱。

（四）又，壳：煮汁饮之，止反胃、消渴。

（五）今有所食生栗，可于热灰中煨之，令才汗出，即啖之，甚破气。不得使通熟，熟即拥气。生即发气。故火煨杀其木气耳。

【注释】

[1] 风水气：病症名。外感风邪、疮毒、水湿导致突发局限性水肿。

[2] 瘅疮毒：瘅指热邪或热气盛。瘅疮毒指由热毒引起的痈疮肿毒等外科和皮肤疾病。

[3] 吴：古地名，中国东部江浙地区的统称，包括今天的浙江钱塘江以北、江苏南部以及上海全境。

## 67. Lizi〔栗子, chestnut, Castaneae Semen〕

Taking raw Lizi〔栗子, chestnut, Castaneae Semen〕can treat the weakness of the waist and feet. Taking the steamed or fried ones will obstruct qi movement. Don't take it when suffering from wind edema[1].

The bark of chestnut tree can resolve heat sore toxin[2].

The following is supplemented by Zhang Ding: It is better to take the sun-dried Lizi〔栗子, chestnut, Castaneae Semen〕as it is effective in descending qi and nourishing the human body. Otherwise, the undried ones contain residual wood qi, which cannot nourish the body. Lizi〔栗子, chestnut, Castaneae Semen〕that grows in Wu[3], large in size while bland in taste, is not as good as that growing in the north. The grinded light coating of it with honey can smooth away wrinkles on the face.

Taking the decoction of its shell can treat regurgitation and consumptive thirst.

It is advisable to roast raw Lizi〔栗子, chestnut, Castaneae Semen〕in hot ash, and eat it when water begins to percolate from its shell. Eating in this way can break the toxin of wood qi, while eating one thoroughly roasted will cause qi stagnation. Raw Lizi〔栗子, chestnut, Castaneae Semen〕can induce wood qi, so roasting it is to resolve the toxin of wood qi.

**【Notes】**

〔1〕wind edema：The name of a disease manifested by the acute and local water swelling caused by external contraction of evil wind, sore-toxin and dampness.

〔2〕heat sore disease："Dan"（瘅）means heat evil and exuberance of heat qi. Heat sore refers to swelling and toxin of welling-abscess and sores caused by heat toxin. It is a dermatosis and surgical disease.

〔3〕Wu：The name of an ancient place. Generally, it refers to the region of Jiangsu and Zhejiang in East China, covering the area from the north of Qiantang River in Zhejiang to the southern part of Jiangsu and the whole Shanghai.

# 68. 覆盆子[1] 平

右主益气轻身,令人发不白。其味甜、酸。五月麦田中得者良。采其子于烈日中晒之,若天雨即烂,不堪收也。江东[2]十月有悬钩子[3],稍小,异形。气味一同。然北地无悬钩子,南方无覆盆子,盖土地殊也。虽两种则不是两种之物,其功用亦相似。

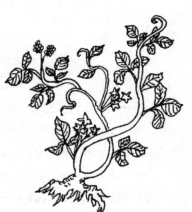

**【注释】**

〔1〕覆盆子:属蔷薇科植物,味甘、酸,性平,有益肾、固精、缩尿、养肝明目之效。

〔2〕江东:古地名,泛指今天的长江以南一带,素以文化繁荣、经济富庶著称。

〔3〕悬钩子:属蔷薇科植物,味酸、甘,性平。全株有补肝健胃、祛风止痛之效。果实有补肾固精之效。

## 68. Fupenzi[1]［覆盆子，palmleaf raspberry fruit，Fructus Rubi］*mild*

Sweet and sour in taste, it is used to replenish qi, relax the body and relieve graying of hair. Those picked from the cornfield in the fifth lunar month are the best. After picking them, dry them in the sun. Exposure to rain will make them rotten and thus unable to be stored. Xuangouzi[2]［悬钩子，raspberry fruit，Rubuscorchorifolius L. F.］produced from Jiangdong[3] in the tenth lunar month has a smaller size and a different shape, but the same flavor with Fupenzi［覆盆子，palmleaf raspberry fruit，Fructus Rubi］. Due to the difference in land and environment, there is no Xuangouzi［悬钩子，raspberry fruit，Rubuscorchorifolius L. F.］in the north and Fupenzi［覆盆子，palmleaf raspberry fruit，Fructus Rubi］does not grow in the south. Despite the different names, they are of the same genus with similar functions.

【Notes】

［1］Fupenzi：The genus of the Rosaceae. Sweet and sour in taste, mild in property, it is effective in tonifying the kidney, securing semen, reducing urination, nourishing the liver and brightening the eyes.

［2］Xuangouzi：The genus of the Rosaceae. It is sweet and sour in taste, and mild in property. The entire plant has effects in nourishing the liver and tonifying the stomach, dispelling wind and relieving pain. Its fruit is effective in tonifying the kidney and securing semen.

［3］Jiangdong：The name of a place in ancient China. Generally, it refers to the region of the south of the Yangtze River, which has always been well renowned for its prosperous culture and economy.

## 69. 芰实(菱实)[1]　平

（一）上主治安中焦，补藏腑气，令人不饥。仙家亦蒸熟曝干作末，和蜜食之休粮。

（二）凡水中之果，此物最发冷气，不能治众疾。（令人藏冷），损阴，令玉茎消衰。

（三）（可少食。多食）令人或腹胀者,以姜、酒一盏,饮即消。含吴茱萸子咽其液亦消。

**【注释】**

〔1〕芰(jì)实(菱实):草本植物菱的果实。鲜品味甘、性凉,有除烦止渴、解酒毒之效。老熟者味甘,性平,能补脾胃。

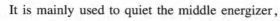

**69. Jishi（Lingshi）[1]〔芰实（菱实）,**
**water caltrop, Trapabispinosa〕** *mild*

It is mainly used to quiet the middle energizer,
replenish qi in the viscera, and enable people to tolerate hunger. The alchemists used to steam it and grind it into powder after sun-drying it, and then take it with honey during inedia.

Among all fruits growing in water, it is the most effective in engendering cold qi, so it can not treat common diseases. Taking it will engender cold qi in the viscera, detriment to yin and flaccid penis.

Taking less is acceptable, but excessive taking may cause abdominal distention which can be relieved by taking a cup of ginger liquor. Holding the seeds of Wuzhuyu〔吴茱萸, medicinal evodia fruit, Fructus Evodiae〕in the mouth and swallowing the saliva can achieve the similar effect.

**【Note】**

〔1〕Jishi（Lingshi）: The fruit of the herbaceous plant-water caltrop. The fresh Jishi（Lingshi）is sweet in taste and cool in property, effective in eliminating vexation, relieving thirst and resolving liquor toxin. The cooked Jishi（Lingshi）is sweet in taste and mild in property, and effective in tonifying the spleen and stomach.

**70. 鸡头子（芡实）[1]** 寒

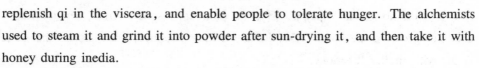

（一）主温[2],治风痹[3],腰脊强直,膝痛。补中焦,益精,强志意,耳目聪明。作粉食之,甚好。此是长生之药。与莲实同食,令小儿不（能）长大,故知长服当亦驻年。

（二）生食动风冷气。可取蒸,于烈日中曝之,其皮壳自开。挼却皮,取人食,甚美。可候皮开,于臼中舂取末。

【注释】

[1]鸡头子(芡实):芡的种仁,属睡莲科水生植物,味甘、涩,性平,有益肾固精、补脾止泻、祛湿止带之效。

[2]温:温病,病名,感受温邪所引起的一类外感急性热病的总称,属广义伤寒的范畴。

[3]风痹:病症名,指因风寒湿侵袭而引起的肢节疼痛或麻木。

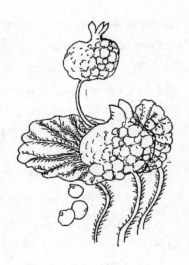

## 70. Jitouzi[1] ( Qianshi ) [鸡头子(芡实), gordaneuryale seed, Semen Euryales] *cold*

It can treat warm diseases[2], wind impediment[3], lumbar spine stiffness and knee pain. It is also effective in tonifying the middle energizer, replenishing essence, and improving memory, thinking, vision and hearing. It is better to make it into powder and take it. It is a medicinal that can prolong life. Taking it with Lianshi [莲实, lotus seed, Nelumbinis Semen] can cause retarded growth in children, which indicates that long-term taking of it can maintain youth.

Taking it raw will stir wind and cold qi. Therefore, it is better to steam it and dry it under the burning sun, which will crack its hull. It is very delicious after removing its hull. It is also acceptable to wait for its hull to crack, grind it into powder in the mortar and take it.

【Notes】

[1] Jitouzi ( Qianshi ): The fruit of the herbaceous plant-Gordon euryale, the genus of the Nymphaeaceae. Sweet in taste, astringent and mild in property, it is effective in supplementing the kidney and astringing essence, fortifying the spleen and checking diarrhea, dispelling dampness and checking vaginal discharge.

[2] warm disease: A general term of the acute external-contraction febrile

diseases caused by the contraction of warm evil. In a broad sense, it falls in the category of cold damage.

[3] wind impediment: A disease referring to the limb joint pain or numbness caused by the invasion of wind, cold and dampness.

# 71. 梅实（乌梅）[1]

（一）食之除闷，安神。乌梅多食损齿。

（二）又，刺在肉中，嚼白梅[2]封之，刺即出。

（三）又，大便不通，气奔[3]欲死：以乌梅十颗置汤中，须臾挼去核，杵为丸，如枣大。内下部，少时即通。

（四）谨按：擘破水渍，以少蜜相和，止渴、霍乱、心腹不安及痢赤。治疟方多用之。

**【注释】**

[1] 梅实（乌梅）：梅的果实，属蔷薇科植物，味酸、涩，性平，有敛肺、涩肠、生津、安蛔之效。

[2] 白梅：梅的未成熟果实，经腌渍而成。

[3] 气奔：病名。指气在人体内如奔跑般移动，伴随皮肤里如波浪声响动，导致游走性瘙痒难忍，即便抓出血也无法缓解。

# 71. Meishi（Wumei）[1] ［梅实（乌梅），
# fruit of Japanese apricot, Fructus Mume］

Taking it can eliminate vexation and quiet spirit, but taking it excessively will damage teeth.

To pull out a thorn deep in the flesh, chew up Baimei[2] ［白梅, candied mume, Mume Fructus Conditus］ and apply it on the wound.

To treat constipation and torturing qi-running[3], soak ten grains of it in hot water for a while, remove the pits, pound them and make into a jujube-sized pill. Put the pill into the anus, and it will not take long to defecate.

The following is supplemented by Zhang Ding: To relieve thirst and treat bloody diarrhea and unquiet heart and abdomen caused by cholera, cut it open, soak it in water, mix it with a bit of honey and then take it. This method is also used often to treat malaria.

**【Notes】**

[1] Meishi (Wumei)：The fruit of Japanese apricot, the genus of the Rosaceae. Sour in taste, astringent and mild in property, it is effective in astringing the lung and the intestines, promoting fluid production and quieting roundworm.

[2] Baimei：The pickled immature fruit of plum.

[3] qi-running：The name of a disease. Qi moves all over the body in the running manner under the skin, making wave-surging sound and resulting in wandering itching which cannot be relieved even by scratching.

# 72. 木　瓜 温

（一）右主治霍乱（呕哕），涩痹风气。

（二）又，顽痹人若吐逆下（利），病转筋不止者，（煮汁饮之甚良）。

（三）脚膝筋急痛，煮木瓜令烂，研作浆粥样，用裹痛处。冷即易，一宿三五度，热裹便瘥。煮木瓜时，入一半酒同煮之。

（四）（谨按）：枝叶煮之饮，亦（治霍乱），去风气，消痰。每欲霍乱时，但呼其名字。亦不可多食，损齿（及骨）。

（五）又，脐下绞痛，可以木瓜一片，桑叶七枚炙，大枣[1]三个中破，以水二大升，煮取半大升，顿服之即（瘥）。

**【注释】**

[1] 大枣：枣的成熟果实，味甘，性温，有补脾和胃、益气生津、养血安神之效。

## 72. Mugua〔木瓜, common floweringqince fruit, Fructus Chaenomelis〕*warm*

It is mainly used to treat cholera complicated by retching and numbness caused by wind impediment.

For people suffering from the intractable disease of wind impediment, taking its decoction is very effective in treating retching counterflow, dysentery and incessant cramp due to diseases.

To treat the acute pain in foot or knee sinews, stew it and grind it into gruel, and wrap it onto the sore spots. Once it gets cold, replace it with hot gruel for three to five times one night. When stewing, add in liquor with half the amount of it.

The following is supplemented by Zhang Ding: Taking the decoction of branches and leaves of its tree can also treat cholera, expel wind evil and resolve phlegm. When suffering from cholera, speak its name out loudly. Do not take too much of it as it can damage the teeth and bones.

To treat the gripping subumbilical pain, take one slice of it, seven leaves of fried Sangye［桑叶, mulberry leaf, Folium Mori］, three Dazao[1]［大枣, Chinese date, Fructus Jujubae］which have been cut open in the middle, decoct them with 2 Sheng of water into half a Sheng, drink the decoction one time, and the pain will be relieved.

【Note】

［1］Dazao: The ripe fruit of Chinese date. Sweet in taste and warm in property, it is effective in tonifying the spleen and harmonizing the stomach, boosting qi and promoting fluid production, nourishing blood and tranquilizing mind.

# 73. 楂 子[1] 平

右多食损齿及损筋。唯治霍乱转筋,煮汁饮之。与木瓜功相似,而小者不如也。昔孔安国[2]不识,而谓(梨)之不藏(者)。今验其形小,况相似。江南将为果子,顿食之。其酸涩也,亦无所益。俗呼为椤梨也。

【注释】

［1］楂子:属蔷薇科植物,味酸、涩,性平,主断痢,去恶心反酸,止酒痰。

［2］孔安国:西汉经学家,孔子十世孙,著有《古文尚书》《论语训解》等作品。

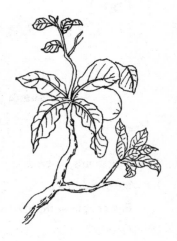

## 73. Zhazi[1]［楂子，Cathy quince，Chaenomelescathayensis Schneid］*mild*

Taking it excessively can damage teeth and sinews，while taking its decoction can treat cholera and cramp. Compared with Mugua［木瓜，common flowering qince fruit，Fructus Chaenomelis］，it has similar effects but is smaller in size and less effective. Kong Anguo[2] once regarded it as low-quality pears as he was not familiar with it. It has now been observed to have similar shape with pears despite the smaller size. People living in the regions of south of the Yangtze River often take it as fruits. It is sour and astringent in taste，and has no tonifying effects. It is commonly known as Xunli（桪梨）.

**［Notes］**

［1］Zhazi：The genus of the Rosaceae. Sour in taste，astringent and mild in property，it is mainly used to treat dysentery，eliminate nausea and acid reflux，and suppress alcoholic phlegm.

［2］Kong Anguo：An expert in studying the Confucian classics of the Western Han Dynasty，the tenth generation descendant of the Confucius，author of the *Gu Wen Shang Shu*［《古文尚书》，*Chinese Ancient Classic*］and *Lun Yu Xun Jie*［《论语训解》，*Interpretation of the Analects of Confucius*］，etc.

## 74. 柿 寒

（一）主通鼻、耳气，补虚劳不足。

（二）谨按：干柿，厚肠胃，温中，健脾胃气，消宿血。

（三）又，红柿：补气，续经脉气。

（四）又，酥柿[1]：涩下焦，健脾胃气，消宿血。作饼及糕，与小儿食，治秋痢。

（五）又，研柿，先煮粥欲熟，即下柿。更三两沸，与小儿饱食，并奶母吃亦良。

（六）又，干柿二斤，酥一斤，蜜半升。先和酥[2]、蜜，铛中消之。下柿，煎十数沸，不津器贮之，每日空腹服三五枚。疗男子、女人脾虚、腹肚薄，食不消化。面上黑点，久服甚良。

【注释】

［1］酥柿：浸渍泡熟的柿子，用温水、冷水、石灰水等脱涩后贮藏。

［2］酥：酪，用牛羊奶凝成的薄皮制造的食物。

## 74. Shi［柿, persimmon, Kaki Fructus］ *cold*

It is mainly used to disinhibit qi in the nose and ears and treat deficiency due to the consumptive disease.

The following is supplemented by Zhang Ding: The dried persimmon can thicken the stomach and intestines, warm the middle, strengthen spleen qi and stomach qi, and dispel the old blood stasis.

The red persimmon can replenish qi and invigorate qi in the meridians.

The preserved persimmon[1] can astringe the lower energizer, strengthen spleen qi and stomach qi and dispel the old blood stasis. Making it into cakes and pastry and feeding infants can treat the autumn dysentery in children.

Grind it into porridge which is going to boil. After boiling two or three times, feed the infants to eat their fill. In the meantime, the breast-feeding mothers taking it can also achieve good effects.

Take 2 Jin of dried persimmon, 1 Jin of milk butter[2] and half a Sheng of honey. Mix and dissolve the milk butter and honey in a pot, add in Shi［柿, persimmon, Kaki Fructus］, decoct them for a dozen times of boiling and store the persimmon in a non-porous container. For both male and female, taking three to five decocted persimmon on an empty stomach every day can treat the spleen deficiency, weak functions of the zang-fu organs and indigestion. Long-term taking of it is effective in removing black macules in the face.

【Notes】

［1］ preserved persimmon: The persimmon preserved after removing the astringency with warm water, cold water or lime water.

［2］ butter: A kind of food made from cow's milk or goat's milk.

# 75. 芋[1] 平

（一）右主宽缓肠胃，去死肌，令脂肉悦泽。

（二）白净者无味，紫色者良，破气。煮汁饮之止渴。十月已后收之，曝干。冬蒸服则不发病，余外不可服。

（三）又，和（鲫鱼、鳢）鱼煮为羹，甚下气，补中焦（良。久食），令人虚，无气力。此物但先肥而已。

（四）又，煮生芋汁，可洗垢腻衣，能洁白（如玉）。

（五）又，煮汁浴之，去身上浮气。浴了，慎风半日许。

【注释】

［1］芋：属天南星科植物，味甘、辛，性平，有益脾胃、调中气、化痰散结之效。

## 75. Yu[1]［芋, taro, Colocasiae Tuber］ *mild*

It is mainly used to harmonize gastrointestinal functions, eliminate necrotic muscles, and moisturize the flesh and skin to be lustrous.

Yu［芋, taro, Colocasiae Tuber］is effective in breaking stagnated qi. Those with white pulp are tasteless and those with purple pulp are better in quality. Taking its decoction can relieve thirst. Harvest it after the tenth lunar month and dry it in the sun. Taking the steamed Yu［芋, taro, Colocasiae Tuber］in winter can prevent diseases, but do not take it in other seasons.

Its soup made with crucian carp and snakehead fish is effective in promoting qi to descend and tonifying the middle energizer. But long-term taking of it will make people weak and fatigued. All its function is only to engender fat.

The decoction of fresh Yu［芋, taro, Colocasiae Tuber］can be used to wash foul clothes and make the clothes as white as the polished jades.

Bathing in its decoction can expel the exterior pathogen. After bath, avoid exposure to wind for half a day.

【Note】

［1］Yu: The genus of the Araceae. Sweet and pungent in taste and mild in property, it is effective in tonifying the spleen and the stomach, harmonizing the middle qi, resolving phlegm and dissipating binds.

# 76. 凫茨(乌芋、荸荠)[1] 寒

下丹石,消风毒,除胸中实热气[2]。可作粉食。明耳目,止渴,消疸黄。若先有冷气,不可食。令人腹胀气满。小儿秋食,脐下当痛。

【注释】

[1] 凫茨:属莎草科植物,味甘,性微寒,有清热化痰、消积、生津止渴和润燥滑肠之效。

[2] 实热气:病症名,又称"实火"。热气指感受外邪或人体机能活动亢进导致阳盛阴衰的热症症候,分为实热和虚热。实热气指阳热亢盛实热证。

# 76. Fuci[1] ( Wuyu, Biqi) [凫茨(乌芋、荸荠), water chestnut, Heleocharitis Cormus] *cold*

It can eliminate the toxin of Danshi, disperse the wind toxin and eliminate the repletion-heat qi[2] in the chest. It can be grinded into powder to take. It can improve hearing and vision, relieve thirst, and treat jaundice. Those who have the cold qi in the body should not take it as it will cause abdominal distention and qi fullness. Infants taking it in autumn will cause the pain below the umbilicus.

【Notes】

[1] Fuci: The genus of the Cyperaceae. Sweet in taste and slightly cold in property, it is effective in clearing heat and transforming phlegm, resolving accumulation, engendering liquid and relieving thirst, moistening dryness and lubricating the intestines.

[2] repletion-heat qi: It is also known as repletion fire. The heat qi is a heat syndrome of exuberance of yang with the decline of yin due to the contraction of external evil or the hyperfunction of the human body. The heat qi can be categorized into repletion heat and deficiency heat. The repletion-heat qi refers to the exuberance of heat yang.

## 77. 茨菰(慈姑)<sup>[1]</sup>

（一）主消渴，下石淋。不可多食。吴人好啖之，令人患脚。

（二）又，发脚气，瘫缓风。损齿，紫黑色。令人失颜色，皮肉干燥。卒食之，令人呕水。

【注释】

［1］茨菰(慈姑)：属泽泻科植物，球茎入药，味苦，性微寒，有解毒利尿、散热消结、强心润肺之效。

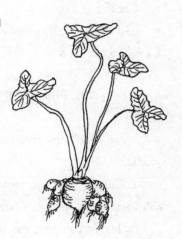

## 77. Cigu<sup>[1]</sup>［茨菰(慈姑)，rhizome of oldworld arrowhead，Sagittariasagittifolia］

It is mainly used to treat the consumptive thirst and stony stranguria. People living in Wu like eating it. Do not eat too much as it will cause weak foot.

Besides weak foot, it may also cause paralysis, damage teeth and make them turn purple-black, make people look pale and make the skin dry. Eating it abruptly will cause the vomiting of water.

【Note】

［1］Cigu：The genus of the Alismaceae. Its corm can be used as medicine. Bitter in taste and slightly cold in property, it is effective in resolving toxin and disinhibiting urine, dissipating heat and binds, strengthening the heart and moistening the lung.

## 78. 枇 杷 温

（一）利五藏，久食亦发热黄。

（二）子：食之润肺，热上膲。若和热炙肉及热面食之，令人患热毒黄病。

（三）（叶）：卒呕哕不止、不欲食。

（四）又，煮汁饮之，止渴。偏理肺及肺风疮<sup>[1]</sup>、胸面上疮。

【注释】

[1] 肺风疮:病症名,又名"肺风"。肺脏感受风毒从而导致皮肤生疮、瘙痒,或面上生疮、鼻头赤烂等。

### 78. Pipa〔枇杷, loquat, Eriobotryae Fructus〕*warm*

It can tonify the five zang-organs, but long-term taking of it will cause heat jaundice.

Taking its fruit can moisten the lung and warm the upper energizer. Taking it with roast meat and hot wheaten food will cause xanthosis due to heat toxin.

Its leaves can treat the incessant retching and anorexia.

Taking its decoction can relieve thirst, rectify the lung and treat the lung wind sore[1] and sore in the chest and face.

【Note】

[1] lung wind sore: A disease referring to contraction of wind toxin in the lung. It causes sores and itching in the skin, sores in the face and ulceration on the bulb of nose.

### 79. 荔　枝[1] 微温

食之通神益智,健气及颜色,多食则发热。

【注释】

[1] 荔枝:属无患子科植物,味甘、酸,性温,可止呕逆、止腹泻,同时有补脑健身、开胃益脾、促进食欲之功效。

### 79. Lizhi[1]〔荔枝, litchee, Litchi Fructus〕*slightly warm*

Taking it can invigorate spirit, promote wisdom, fortify qi and luster the facial expression. Taking it excessively will cause heat effusion.

【Note】

[1] Lizhi: The genus of the Sapindaceae. Sweet and sour in taste and warm in property, it can treat retching counterflow and diarrhea. It is also effective in

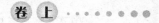

tonifying the brain and strengthening the body, stimulating and increasing the appetite and tonifying the spleen.

# 80. 柑子（乳柑子）[1] 寒

（一）堪食之，其皮不任药用。初未霜时，亦酸。及得霜后，方即甜美。故名之曰甘。

（二）利肠胃热毒，下丹石，（止暴）渴。食多令人肺燥[2]，冷中，发流癖[3]病也。

【注释】

［1］柑子（乳柑子）：属芸香科植物，味甘、酸，性凉，有清热生津、醒酒利尿、疏肝理气等功效。

［2］肺燥：病症名，指外感燥邪、耗伤肺津、肺卫失和导致干咳痰少、鼻咽口舌干燥等症状。

［3］流癖：病名，又称"疝癖"。因气血不和、经络阻滞、食积寒凝，导致脐腹或胁肋部有条状筋块扛起，平时寻摸不见，痛时摸之才觉有物。

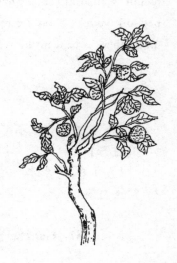

# 80. Ganzi[1]（Ruganzi）［柑子（乳柑子），citrus, Materia Medica Ganzi］cold

It is edible but its pericarp can not be used as medicine. It tastes sour before the frost falls, and turns sweet after getting frosted. For that reason, it has the word "gan"［甘, means sweet in Chinese］in its names.

It can disinhibit the heat toxin in the stomach and intestines, eliminate the toxin of Danshi and relieve the extreme thirst. Excessive taking will cause lung dryness[2], engender cold qi in the middle energizer, and cause strings and aggregations[3].

【Notes】

［1］Ganzi：The genus of the Rutaceae. Sweet and sour in taste and cool in property, it is effective in clearing heat and engendering liquid, dispelling the effects of liquor and disinhibiting urine, coursing the liver and rectifying qi.

〔2〕lung dryness：A disease referring to the contraction of dryness evil which impairs the lung liquids and defense and thus causes symptoms such as dry cough with scant phlegm，dryness of nose，throat，mouth and tongue，etc.

〔3〕strings and aggregations：A disease in the umbilical region or the rib-side region with strings and aggregations due to qi and blood，obstruction of channels and network vessels，food accumulation or cold congealment．It can not be felt easily unless there is pain in the region.

# 81. 甘　蔗[1]

主补气，兼下气。不可共酒食，发痰。
【注释】
〔1〕甘蔗：属禾本科植物，以秆、汁入药，味甘、涩，性平，有消热、生津、下气、润燥之效。

## 81. Ganzhe[1]〔甘蔗，**sugar cane**，**Sacchari Caulis**〕

It is mainly used to replenish qi and promot qi to descend．Do not take it with liquor as it will engender phlegm.
【Note】
〔1〕Ganzhe：The genus of the Graminaceae．Its stalk and juice can be used as medicine．Sweet in taste，astringent and mild in property，it is effective in expelling heat，promoting fluid production，descending qi and moistening dryness.

# 82. 石蜜（乳糖）[1] 寒

（一）右心腹胀热，口干渴。波斯[2]者良。注少许于目中，除去热膜[3]，明目。蜀川[4]者为次。今东吴[5]亦有，并不如波斯。此皆是煎甘蔗汁及牛乳汁，煎则细白耳。

（二）又，和枣肉及巨胜人[6]作末为丸，每食后含一丸如李核大，咽之津，润肺气，助五藏津。

【注释】
〔1〕石蜜（乳糖）：甘蔗汁或白糖经过太阳曝晒或熬制而成的块状固体，味

甘,性寒,有润肺生津、止渴、滋阴、除口臭、解毒之功效。

　　[2] 波斯:伊朗的古名。

　　[3] 热膜:热毒郁结形成的眼结膜病态增生,即眼翳。

　　[4] 蜀川:古地名,指蜀地,今天的四川省。

　　[5] 东吴:古地名,三国时期吴国居于三国之东,故称"东吴",后泛指今天的江苏南部、浙江、安徽南部地区。

　　[6] 巨胜人:味甘,性平,主治内脏损伤、身体虚弱消瘦,有滋补五脏、润燥滑肠、补益气力、滋养肝肾之效。

## 82. Shimi (Rutang)[1] [石蜜(乳糖), Chinese honey bee, Apis] *cold*

It is mainly used to treat distention and fullness in the heart and abdomen and relieve thirst and dry mouth. That produced in Persia[2] is the best. Dripping a bit of it into the eyes can remove the heat membrane[3] and improve vision. That produced in Shuchuan[4] takes the second place in regard to quality. Dongwu[5] also produces it, but not as good as that of Persia. Decoct Ganzhezhi [甘蔗汁, sugar cane juice, Sacchari Caulis Succus] and cow milk until it looks fine and white, and then Shimi [石蜜, Chinese honey bee, Apis] is produced.

Grind it with Dazao [大枣, Chinese date, Fructus Jujubae] and Jushengren[6] [巨胜人, black sesame, Sesami Semen Nigrum] into powder and make pills. After meal, hold a pill in size of the plum kernel in the mouth. Swallowing the saliva can moisten lung qi and supplement the fluids in the five zang-organs.

【Notes】

[1] Shimi (Rutang): Solid block decocted or dried out of the sugar cane juice or white sugar. Sweet in taste and cold in property, it is effective in moistening the lung and engendering liquids, relieving thirst, nourishing yin, removing fetid mouth odor, resolving toxin, etc.

[2] Persia: The old name of Iran.

[3] heat membrane: It is a disease called pathological hyperplasia of conjunction caused by binding depression of heat toxin, also known as pterygium.

[4] Shuchuan: The old name of Sichuan Province.

[5] Dongwu: The name of an ancient place. During the Three Kingdoms

Period, the Wu State was located to the east（Dong，"东"）of the three states，giving it the name Dongwu. It refers to the region covering the south of Jiangsu Province，Zhejiang Province，and the south of Anhui Province in today's China.

［6］Jushengren：Sweet in taste and mild in property，it is mainly used to treat the injury of internal organs，vacuity and emaciation. It is effective in tonifying the five zang-organs，moistening dryness and lubricating the intestines，supplementing the body strength，and tonifying the liver and kidney.

# 83. 沙　糖[1] 寒

（一）右功体与石蜜同也。多食令人心痛。养三虫，消肌肉，损牙齿，发疳䘌[2]。不可多服之。

（二）又，不可与鲫鱼同食，成疳虫。

（三）又，不与葵[3]同食，生流澼。

（四）又，不可共笋食之，（使）笋不消，成症病心腹痛。（身）重不能行履。

**【注释】**

［1］沙糖：即砂糖，指甘蔗汁经过太阳曝晒或简单炼制后的固体原始蔗糖，味甘，性寒，与石蜜功效相同。

［2］疳䘌：即鼻疳，病名，湿热邪毒上犯或血虚生风化燥而致的以鼻前孔及其附近皮肤红肿、糜烂、渗液、结痂、灼痒或皲裂为主要特征的鼻部疾病，常反复发作，经久不愈。

［3］葵：古代蔬菜名。又称"葵菜"或"冬苋菜"，有清热利湿之效。

## 83. Shatang[1]［沙糖，granulated sugar，Saccharon Granulatum］ *cold*

It has the similar functions and size with Shimi［石蜜，Chinese honey bee，Apis］. Excessive taking of it will cause pain in the heart，engender three kinds of worms，weaken muscles，damage teeth and cause Ganni[2]. So do not take it excessively.

Do not take it with crucian carp as it will cause Gan worm.

Do not take it with the courled mallow[3] as it will cause strings and aggregations.

Do not take it with the bamboo shoot as it will cause the indigestion of bamboo shoots, which will make into accumulation lump and thus cause pain in the heart and abdomen and heavy body with difficulty to walk.

【Notes】

[1] Shatang: Also known as Shatang（砂糖）, solid cane sugar made from drying in the sun or roughly refining the sugar cane juice. Sweet in taste and cold in property, it has the similar functions with Shimi［石蜜, Chinese honey bee, Apis］.

[2] Ganni: It is also called Bigan（鼻疳）, nasal vestibulitis in the Western medicine, which is a disease characterized by redness, swelling, ulceration, exudation, crusting, cracking and burning itching in the nasal vestibule and the skin around it. It is caused by invading the upper body by the damp heat evil-toxin or dryness formation by blood deficiency engendering wind and it is frequently recurrent and difficult to be cured.

[3] courled mallow: A vegetable which is effective in clearing heat and disinhibiting dampness.

# 84. 桃人（仁）  温

（一）杀三虫,止心痛。

（二）又,女人阴中生疮,如虫咬、疼痛者,可生捣叶,绵裹内阴中,日三、四易,瘥。亦煮汁洗之。今案:煮皮洗之良。

（三）又,三月三日收花晒干,杵末,以水服二钱匕。小儿半钱,治心腹痛。

（四）又,秃疮[1]:收未开花阴干,与桑椹赤者,等分作末,以猪脂和。先用灰汁洗去疮痂,即涂药。

（五）又云,桃能发诸丹石,不可食之。生者尤损人。

（六）又,白毛:主恶鬼邪气。胶亦然。

（七）又,桃符及奴[2]:主精魅邪气。符,煮汁饮之;奴者,丸、散服之。

（八）桃人:每夜嚼一颗,和蜜涂手、面良。

【注释】

[1] 秃疮:又称"白秃疮""癞头疮""头疮",是多发生在头部的一种癣。其特征为脱落白屑,久则毛发折断脱落成秃疮,愈后毛发常可再生。

[2] 奴:桃奴,即"瘰桃干""阴桃子""气桃子",指未经受精所结晚熟的小

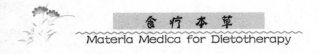
桃,有止痛、止汗之效。

## 84. Taoren［桃人(仁)，peach seed，Semen Persicae］*warm*

It can kill three kinds of worms and relieve the pain in heart.

To treat the genital sore with pain like bitten by worms, smash the fresh peach leaves, wrap it in Mian［绵，silk floss，Bombycis Lana］and put it into the vagina. Change it for three or four times a day and then the sore will be cured. It is also advisable to wash the vagina with its decoction. Supplement nowadays: Washing the vagina with the decoction of the bark of peach trees can achieve good effects.

On the third day of the third lunar month, harvest the peach blossoms, dry them, pound them into powder and take 2 Qianbi of the powder with water. Infants taking half a Qianbi can treat the pain in heart and abdomen.

To treat bald scalp sore[1], harvest the not-blossoming flower buds and dry them in the shade, smash them with the same amount of ripe Sangshen［桑葚，mulberry，Mori Fructus］and mix them up with Zhuzhi［猪脂，pork lard，Suis Adeps］. Apply it on the infected part after rinsing off scabs with plant ash water.

Peach can cause the toxin of Danshi, so those who take Danshi should not take it. The unripe peaches are particularly harmful.

The white peach fuzz can expel severe pathogenic factors like ghost and eliminate evil qi. Taojiao［桃胶，peach resin，Persicae Resina］has the similar functions.

The peach wood and Taonu[2] can expel severe pathogenic factors like ghost and eliminate evil qi. To achieve that effect, take the decoction of the peach wood, and take the pills or powder made of Taonu.

Chew one Taoren［桃人(仁)，peach seed，Semen Persicae］, mix it with honey and apply it on the hands and face every night. This method can nourish the skin.

【Note】

［1］bald scalp sore: It is also known as white bald scalp sore. It is a type of head dermatoses, commonly caused by unclean barber tools or infection from combs or hats. Crusts first appear on the head, causing unbearable pruritus and then develop

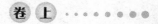

to a large scale of contagious sores, followed by hair loss and baldness over time. But the hair can regenerate when the sores are healed.

［2］Taonu：Also known as "Bietaogan"（瘪桃干）, "Yintaozi"（阴桃子）or "Qitaozi"（气桃子）. It refers to the later maturing unfertilized pigmy fruit of peach, which is effective in relieving pain and checking sweating.

## 85. 樱　桃 热

（一）益气，多食无损。

（二）又云，此名"樱"，非桃也。不可多食，令人发暗风[1]。

（三）温。多食有所损。令人好颜色，美志。此名"樱桃"，俗名"李桃"，亦名"奈桃"者是也。甚补中益气，主水谷痢[2]，止泄精。

（四）东行根：疗寸白、蚘虫。

【注释】

［1］暗风：病症名，是一种与内风相似，由脏腑功能失调引致风阳上亢的疾病。主要症状是头晕眼黑、不辨东西。发病过程缓慢，往往在不知不觉中逐步发病。

［2］水谷痢：病症名。因脾胃气虚，不能消化水谷导致腹泻腹痛，泻下物中有不消化的食物。

## 85. Yingtao［樱桃, cherry, Pruni Pseudocerasi Fructus］*hot*

It can replenish qi, so eating a lot does no harm to our body.

It is called "Yingtao", but not a kind of peach（Tao, "桃"）. Do not take it excessively, otherwise it will cause latent wind[1].

It is also warm in property. Excessive taking of it is harmful. It can luster facial expression and invigorate spirit. Its popular name is Litao（李桃）, also known as Naitao（奈桃）. It is quite effective in tonifying the middle and replenishing qi, so it is mainly used to treat grain and water dysentery[2] and seminal discharge.

The eastward roots of cherry trees can expel tapeworms and roundworms in the stomach.

【Notes】

［1］latent wind: A disease similar to the internal wind, caused by the dysfunction of zang-fu organs complicated with the ascendant hyperactivity of wind yang. The main symptoms are dizzy head and dim vision. It develops slowly and gradually before it is recognized.

［2］grain and water dysentery: A disease caused by spleen-stomach qi deficiency. The indigestion of grain and water causes diarrhea and abdominal pain, with indigested food in the excrement.

# 86. 杏 热

（一）主咳逆上气,金创,惊痫[1],心下烦热,风(气)头痛。

（二）面皯者,取人去皮,捣和鸡子白。夜卧涂面,明早以暖清酒洗之。

（三）人患卒瘖,取杏人三分,去皮尖熬,(捣作脂。)别杵桂(心)一分,和如泥。取李核大,绵裹含,细细咽之,日五夜三。

（四）谨按:心腹中结伏气:杏人、橘皮、桂心、诃梨勒[2]皮为丸,空心服三十丸,无忌。

（五）又,烧令烟尽,去皮,以乱发裹之,咬于所患齿下,其痛便止。熏诸虫出,并去风便瘥。重者不过再服。

（六）又,烧令烟尽,研如泥,绵裹内女人阴中,治虫疽。

【注释】

［1］惊痫:病名,因受惊而致。病症轻者身热面赤,睡眠不安,时常惊醒;重者眼往上翻,身体强直,甚至全身抽搐。

［2］诃梨勒:即柯子,常绿乔木,果实可入药,有涩肠止泻、敛肺止咳、利咽开音之效。

## 86. Xing［杏, apricot, Pruni Armeniacae］*hot*

It is mainly used to treat cough with dyspnea and upward counterflow of qi, metal injury, fright epilepsy[1], vexing heat in epigastrium, and headache due to the wind qi.

To treat the withered facial expression and remove the black macules in the face, pound the peeled apricot seeds, mix them with egg white, apply the mixture on the face before going to sleep, and wash it off with warm clear liquor in the next morning.

To treat the sudden aphonia, remove 3 Fen of seed coat and germ of Xingren ［杏人, apricot seed, Semen Armeniacae］, decoct them and pound them until the oil comes out. Pound 1 Fen of Guixin ［桂心, shaved cinnamon bark, Cinnamomi Cortex Rasus］ and mix it with the apricot seed paste. Take the mixed paste in size of a plum kernel and wrap it with Mian ［绵, silk floss, Bombycis Lana］. Put it in the mouth and swallow the saliva. Do that for five times in the day and three times in the evening.

The following is supplemented by Zhang Ding. To treat the stagnation of latent qi in the heart and abdomen, make pills with Xingren ［杏人, apricot seed, Semen Armeniacae］, Jupi ［橘皮, tangerine peel, Citri Reticulatae Pericarpium］, Guixin ［桂心, shaved cinnamon bark, Cinnamomi Cortex Rasus］ and peel of Kelile[2] ［诃梨勒, chebule, Chebulae Fructus］, and take thirty pills on an empty stomach, without any dietary contraindication.

Burn Xingren ［杏人, apricot seed, Semen Armeniacae］ until there is no smoke any more, peel it, wrap it with reckless hair and put it underneath the sick tooth. Then the toothache will be relieved. When all the worms and the wind evil are smoked out, the toothache is healed. Even the severe patient just need to do it one more time.

To treat the worm abscess, burn Xingren ［杏人, apricot seed, Semen Armeniacae］ until there is no smoke anymore, pound it into paste, wrap it in Mian ［绵, silk floss, Bombycis Lana］ and put it in the vagina.

**［Notes］**

［1］fright epilepsy: A disease caused by fright. The patients suffering from it mildly have generalized fever, red face, unquiet sleep and frequent awakening from night. Those severe cases have upturned eyes, rigid body, even convulsion of the whole body.

［2］Kelile: Also known as Kezi (柯子), a type of evergreen tree. Its fruit can be used as medicine, and it is effective in astringing the intestines and checking diarrhea, astringing lung and relieving cough, disinhibiting the throat and restoring the voice.

## 87. 石 榴 温

（一）实：主谷利、泄精。

（二）（东行根：疗）疣虫白虫。

（三）按经：久食损齿令黑。其皮炙令黄，捣为末，和枣肉为丸，（空腹）日服三十丸，后以饭押，（日二服）。断赤白痢。

（四）又，久患赤白痢，肠肚绞痛：以醋石榴一个，捣令碎，布绞取汁，空腹顿服之立止。

（五）又，其花叶阴干，捣为末，和铁丹服之。一年白发尽黑，益面红色。仙家重此，不尽书其方。

## 87. Shiliu〔石榴，pomegranate，Granati Fructus〕*warm*

Its fruit is mainly used to treat grain dysentery and seminal discharge.

The eastward root can expel roundworm and tapeworm.

The following is supplemented by Zhang Ding: Long-term taking of it can damage and blacken the teeth. To treat the red and white dysentery, fry its rind until it turns yellow, grind it into powder, make it into pills with Zaorou〔枣肉，jujube flesh, Jujubae Pericarpium〕, take thirty pills every day on an empty stomach and then take meal to ease its side effect. Take it twice a day.

To treat the enduring red and white dysentery and the gripping pain in the intestines and abdomen, pound a Suanshiliu〔酸石榴，sour pomegranate, Granati Fructus Acidus〕, wrap it in the cloth to wring out juice, take all the juice one time on an empty stomach, and then the dysentery will be cured right away.

Dry its flowers and leaves in the shade, pound them into powder and take it with colcothar. After one-year taking, the white hair will all turn black, and the complexion will become ruddy. The alchemists valued this formula, so they did not let the public know in details.

## 88. 梨 寒

（一）除客热，止心烦。不可多食。

（二）又，卒咳嗽，以冻梨一颗刺作五十孔，每孔中内以椒一粒。以面裹于热灰中煨，令极熟，出停冷，去椒食之。

（三）又方，梨去核，内酥蜜，面裹烧令熟。食之大良。

（四）又方，去皮，割梨肉，内于酥中煎之。停冷食之。

（五）又，捣汁一升，酥一两，蜜一两，地黄[1]汁一升，缓火煎，细细含咽。凡治嗽，皆须待冷，喘息定后方食。热食之，反伤矣，令嗽更极不可救。如此者，可作羊肉汤饼，饱食之，便卧少时。

（六）又，胸中痞塞、热结者，可多食好生梨即通。

（七）（又云），卒暗风，失音不语者，生捣（梨）汁一合，顿服之。日再服，止。

（八）金疮及产妇不可食，大忌。

**【注释】**

[1] 地黄：中药材，玄参科植物地黄的块根，味甘，性寒，有滋阴补肾、养血补血、强心利尿等功效。

## 88. Li［梨，pear，Pyri Fructus］*cold*

It can eliminate visiting heat and check vexation, but do not eat it excessively.

To treat the sudden cough, prick fifty holes in a frozen pear, put a grain of pepper in each hole, wrap the pear with flour and roast it in hot ash. When it is well done, cool it, remove the peppers and eat it.

Another formula：Remove its kernel, put in butter and honey, wrap it with flour and bake it thoroughly. Eating it can achieve very desirable effects.

Another formula：Remove the peel, cut off the flesh, put it in the butter, decoct it and eat it when it gets cool.

To treat cough, crush it to extract 1 Sheng of juice, decoct it over a low flame with 1 Liang of butter, 1 Liang of honey and 1 Sheng of Dihuang[1]［地黄，Rehmannia root, Radix Rehmanniae］juice, and swallow the decoction slowly. It is necessary to cool it and then take it when the patient stops panting. Taking the hot decoction is harmful and will exacerbate the cough. In that case, it is advisable to make some mutton soup and cakes and lie on bed for a while after taking them.

To treat glomus blockage and heat bind in the chest, eat more good-quality fresh Li [梨, pear, Pyri Fructus].

To treat the sudden latent wind syndrome and the loss of voice, crush out 1 Ge of pear juice and take it one time. Take it twice a day, and then the disease will be cured.

The metal-injury patients and the puerperae should not eat it as it is a definite taboo of food for them.

【Note】

[1] Dihuang: The root of Dihuang which is the genus of the Scrophulariaceae. Sweet in taste and cold in property, it is effective in nourishing yin and tonifying the kidney and blood, strengthening the heart and disinhibiting urine.

# 89. 林 檎[1] 温

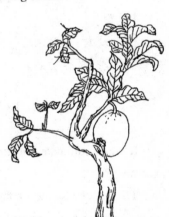

（一）主谷痢、泄精。东行根治白虫蛲虫。

（二）主止消渴。好睡，不可多食。

（三）又，林檎味苦涩、平，无毒。食之闭百脉。

【注释】

[1] 林檎：又名"花红""沙果"，属蔷薇科植物，其果实可食，有止渴、化滞、涩精之效。

## 89. Linqin[1] [林檎, **Chinese crabapple**, **Mali Asiaticae Fructus**] *warm*

Linqin [林檎, Chinese crabapple, Mali Asiaticae Fructus] is mainly used to treat grain dysentery and seminal discharge. The eastward root can expel whiteworm and roundworm.

It is effective in quenching consumptive thirst. Do not take it excessively as it will cause somnolence.

It is bitter and astringent in taste, and mild and non-toxic in property. Taking it may obstruct all vessels.

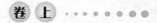

【Note】

［1］Linqin：Also known as Huahong（花红）or Shaguo（沙果），the genus of the Rosaceae. Its fruit is edible. It is effective in relieving thirst, resolving stagnation and astringing essence.

## 90. 李 平

（一）主女人卒赤、白下：取李树东面皮，去外皮，炙令黄香。以水三升，煮汁去滓服之，日再验。

（二）谨按：生李亦去骨节间劳热，不可多食之。临水食之，令人发痰疟[1]。

（三）又，牛李[2]：有毒。煮汁使浓，含之治蜃齿。脊骨有疳虫，可后灌此汁，更空腹服一盏。

（四）其子中人：主鼓胀。研和面作饼子，空腹食之，少顷当泻矣。

【注释】

［1］痰疟：病名，较重型疟疾，临床表现为发作时寒热交作、热多寒少、头痛眩晕、痰多呕逆、脉弦滑，类似脑型疟疾。

［2］牛李：鼠李的古名。

## 90. Li［李，plum，Pruni Salicinae Fructus］ *mild*

To treat the sudden red and white vaginal discharge, take the eastward bark of plum trees and remove the exterior raw bark, roast it until it turns yellow and smells fragrant, decoct it with 3 Sheng of water, remove the dregs and take it. Taking it twice a day will achieve effects.

The following is supplemented by Zhang Ding：Unripe Li［李，plum，Pruni Salicinae Fructus］can eliminate the bone taxation heat, but do not eat it excessively. Eating it with water will cause phlegm malaria[1].

Niuli[2]［牛李，davurian buckthorn fruit，Fructus Rhamni Davuricae］is toxic in property. Decocting it and holding the thick juice in mouth can treat the tooth decay. The patients with Gan worm eating into spines can first apply the juice in enema and then take 1 Zhan of the juice on an empty stomach.

The kernel of Niuli［牛李，davurian buckthorn fruit，Fructus Rhamni

Davuricae〕can treat tympanites. Grind it into powder, make cakes with flour, eat the cakes on an empty stomach, and it doesn't take long time to drain the accumulated food.

【Notes】

〔1〕phlegm malaria：One severe type of malaria. Its clinical manifestations include alternating cold and fever, more fever than cold, headache and dizziness, copious phlegm and retching counterflow, wiry and rolling pulse. It is similar to the cerebral malaria.

〔2〕Niuli：The old name of Shuli〔鼠李, davurian buckthorn fruit, Fructus Rhamni Davuricae〕.

# 91. 羊(杨)梅 温

（一）右主(和)藏腑，调腹胃，除烦愦，消恶气，去痰实。

（二）(亦)不可多食，损人(齿及)筋(也)，然(甚能)断下痢。

（三）又，烧为灰，(亦)断下痢。其味酸美，小有胜白梅。

（四）又，取干者，常含一枚，咽其液，亦通利五藏，下少气。

（五）若多食，损人筋骨。甚酸之物，是土地使然。若南人北，杏亦不食。北人南，梅亦不噉。皆是地气郁蒸，令烦愦，好食斯物也。

## 91. Yangmei〔羊(杨)梅, bayberry, Myricae Fructus〕 *warm*

It is mainly used to harmonize the zang-fu organs, regulate the intestine and stomach, eliminate vexation, disperse the malign qi and dissipate the phlegm-heat retention.

Do not take it excessively as it may damage the teeth, sinews and bones. But it is very effective in treating dysentery.

The ash of burnt Yangmei〔杨梅, bayberry, Myricae Fructus〕can also treat dysentery. It is sour and palatable in taste, slightly superior to that of Baimei〔白梅, candied mume, Mume Fructus Conditus〕.

Frequently hold a grain of dry Yangmei〔杨梅, bayberry, Myricae Fructus〕in the mouth and swallow the saliva, which can disinhibit the five zang-organs and slightly promote qi to descend.

Excessive taking of it will damage the sinews and bones. Its sour taste is due to the geographical difference. The southerners going to the north are not adaptable to the sourness of Xing〔杏, apricot, Pruni Armeniacae〕 but the northerners going to the south are favorable of the sourness of Yangmei〔杨梅, bayberry, Myricae Fructus〕. In the south, the depressing steaming earth qi causes vexation easily, which explains why the people living there like eating Yangmei〔杨梅, bayberry, Myricae Fructus〕.

## 92. 胡　桃[1] 平

（一）右（卒）不可多食，动痰（饮）。

（二）案经:除去风,润脂肉,令人能食。不得多食之,计日月,渐渐服食。通经络气,（润）血脉,黑人鬓发、毛落再生也。

（三）又,烧至烟尽,研为泥,和胡粉[2]为膏。拔去白发,敷之即黑毛发生。

（四）又,仙家压油,和詹香[3]涂黄发,便黑如漆,光润。

（五）初服日一颗,后随日加一颗。至廿颗,定得骨细肉润。

（六）又方,（能瘥）一切痔病。

（七）案经:动风,益气,发痼疾。多吃不宜。

【注释】

［1］胡桃:俗称"核桃",植物胡桃的种仁,味甘,性平,有润肺补肾、止咳平喘、润燥滑肠之效。

［2］胡粉:矿物铅加工制成的铅粉,有败毒抗癌、杀虫疗疮、祛瘀止血之效。

［3］詹香:又名"必栗香",见李时珍《本草纲目》。

## 92. Hutao[1]〔胡桃, walnut, Juglandis Semen〕 *mild*

Do not take it excessively as it will cause phlegm-fluid retention.

The following is supplemented by Zhang Ding: It can expel the wind evil, moisten the skin and promote appetite, but do not take too much one time. Instead, take it gradually over time, which can dredge qi of the collaterals, moisten the blood vessels, blacken and boost hair.

Burn it until there is no smoke anymore, grind it into cream and make it into paste with Hufen[2][胡粉, processed galenite, Galenitum Praeparatum]. Pluck the white hair and apply the paste to the head, and then black hair will regrow.

The alchemists used to grind it to extract oil, mix the oil with Zhanxiang[3] and apply it to the yellowing hair which will make the hair turn black and sheen.

Take one on the first day and one more on the following day until taking twenty a day, when you will surely get dense bones and smooth skin.

It can treat all kinds of hemorrhoids.

The following is supplemented by Zhang Ding: It can stir wind, replenish qi and cause intractable diseases; therefore, it is unsuitable to take it excessively.

【Notes】

[1] Hutao: Commonly known as Hetao (核桃). The seed of Hutao is the genus of the Juglandaceae. Sweet in taste and mild in property, it is effective in moistening the lung and tonifying the kidney, relieving cough and dyspnea, moistening dryness and clearing the intestines.

[2] Hufen: Powder processed from galenite. It is effective in vanquishing toxins and curing cancers, killing worms and healing sores, dispelling stasis and stanching bleeding.

[3] Zhanxiang: Also known as Bilixiang (必栗香), it is probably Huaxiangshu [化香树, platycarya, Platycarya Strobilacea Sieb. et Zucc.]. See *Ben Cao Gang Mu* [《本草纲目》 *Compendium of Materia Medica*] by Li Shizhen.

# 93. 藤梨[1](猕猴桃) 寒

右主下丹石,利五藏。其熟时,收取瓤和蜜煎作煎。服之去烦热,止消渴。久食发冷气,损脾胃。

【注释】

[1] 藤梨:又称"羊桃""猕猴桃""棠梨",猕猴桃科植物猕猴桃的果实,口感酸甜,含丰富的矿物质、氨基酸、维生素C、有机物、葡萄糖等,有降低血压、提升免疫力等功效。

## 93. Tengli[1] (Mihoutao) [藤梨(猕猴桃), Chinese gooseberry, Actinidiae Chinensis Fructus] *cold*

It is mainly used to eliminate the toxin of Danshi and benefit the five zang-organs. When it gets ripe, mix its flesh with honey and decoct them into paste. Taking the paste can eliminate the vexing heat and treat the consumptive thirst. Long-term taking will engender the cold qi and damage the spleen and stomach.

【Note】

[1] Tengli: Also known as Yangtao (羊桃), Mihoutao (猕猴桃) or Tangli (棠梨), the fruit of Actinidia chinensis Planch (the genus of the Actinidiaceae). It is sour and sweet in taste, rich in mineral substance, amino acid, Vitamin C, organism, glucose, etc. It is effective in lowering blood pressure, improving immunity, etc.

## 94. 柰[1]

益心气,主补中膲诸不足气,和脾。卒患食后气不通,生捣汁服之。

【注释】

[1] 柰(nài):苹果的一个品种,味甘,性寒,有生津止渴、益气和脾之效。

## 94. Nai[1] [柰, apple, Mali Pumulae Fructus]

It can tonify the heart qi, supplement the insufficient qi of the middle energizer and harmonize the spleen. To treat suffering from the sudden qi stagnation after taking meals, pound it into juice and take it.

【Notes】

[1] Nai: One variety of apple. Sweet in taste and cold in property, it is effective in engendering liquid and relieving thirst, replenishing qi and harmonizing the spleen.

# 95. 橄榄(橄榄)[1]

主鯸鱼毒,(煮)汁服之。中此鱼肝、子毒,人立死,惟此木能解。出岭南[2]山谷。大树阔数围,实长寸许。其子先生者向下,后生者渐高。至八月熟,蜜藏极甜。

**【注释】**

[1] 橄榄(橄榄):橄榄科乔木植物,其果实味酸甘,性平,有清热解毒、利咽化痰、生津止渴、除烦醒酒之效。

[2] 岭南:五岭(越城岭、都庞岭、萌渚岭、骑田岭、大庾岭)以南的地区,大致分布在广西东部至广东东部和湖南、江西交界处。

## 95. Ganyan (Ganlan)[1] [橄榄(橄榄), olive, Fructus Canarii Albi]

Taking its decoction can resolve the toxin of globefish. The toxin in the liver and roe of globefish can kill people right away, which can only be resolved by it. It grows in the valleys in the south of the Five Ridges[2]. Its trunk can be so thick that it can only be encircled by several people joining their hands, and its fruit can be as long as about 1 Cun. The first growing fruits are at the lower parts of the branches, and the later growing fruits are gradually rising. The fruit gets ripe in the eighth lunar month, and it is especially sweet when preserved in honey.

**【Notes】**

[1] Ganyan (Ganlan): Macrophanerophytes of the Burseraceae. Its fruit is sour and sweet in taste and mild in property. It is effective in clearing heat and resolving toxin, disinhibiting the throat and resolving phlegm, engendering liquid and relieving thirst, eliminating vexation and restoring soberness.

[2] The south of the Five Ridges: The Five Ridges refer to the mountain ridges including Yuechen mountains and Dupang mountains, Mengzhu mountains, Qitian mountains and Dayu mountians. The south of the Five Ridges refers to the southern area of them, ranging from the east of Guangxi Province to the east of Guangdong Province and the junction of the provinces of Hunan and Jiangxi.

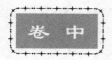

# Volume 2

## 96. 麝 香

（一）作末服之，辟诸毒热，煞蛇毒，除惊怪[1]恍惚。蛮人常食，似獐肉而腥气。蛮人云：食之不畏蛇毒故也。

（二）脐中有香[2]，除百病，治一切恶气痘病[3]。研了，以水服之。

【注释】

［1］惊怪：因为受到惊吓而患的疾病。

［2］古代人以为麝香从麝鹿的肚脐分泌。

［3］痘病：具有传染性和病程长的慢性病。

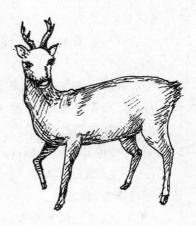

## 96. Shexiang［麝香, abelmusk, Moschus］

Ground into powder, it can repel various toxic heat, resolve snake toxins and treat convulsion[1] and spirit abstraction. Savages often ate the meat of musk deer, tasting like roe meat and smelling fishy. They said that they were not afraid of snake toxins because of eating the meat of the musk deer.

With fragrance in the navel of the musk deer[2], known as abelmusk, Shexiang［麝香, abelmusk, Moschus］ has a clinical effect on all diseases, especially treating all infixation diseases[3] caused by the malign qi. Grind it into powder and take it with water.

【Notes】

［1］convulsion: A mental disease caused by shock.

［2］with fragrance in the navel of the musk deer: The ancients thought that the abelmusk was a kind of fragrance secreted from the navel of the musk deer.

［3］ infixation disease：A chronic infectious disease lasting a long time.

# 97. 牛

（一）牛者稼穑之资，不多屠杀。自死者，血脉已绝，骨髓已竭，不堪食。黄牛发药动病，黑牛尤不可食。黑牛尿及屎，只入药。

（二）又，头、蹄：下热风[1]，患冷人不可食。

（三）肝：治痢。又，肝醋煮食之，治瘦。

（四）肚：主消渴，风眩[2]，补五脏，以醋煮食之。

（五）肾：主补肾。

（六）髓：安五藏，平三焦，温中。久服增年。以酒送之。黑牛髓，和地黄汁、白蜜等分，作煎服之，治瘦病。恐是牛脂也。

（七）粪：主霍乱，煮饮之。乌牛粪为上。又小儿夜啼，取干牛粪如手大，安卧席下，勿令母知，子、母俱吉。

（八）又，妇人无乳汁，取牛鼻作羹，空心食之。不过三两日，有汁下无限。若中年壮盛者，食之良。

（九）又，宰之尚不堪食，非论自死者。其牛肉取三斤，烂切，将啖解槽咬人恶马，只两啖后，颇甚驯良。若三五顿后，其马狞狚不堪骑。十二月勿食，伤神。

【注释】

［1］热风：病症名，受风热侵袭所引发的病变。

［2］风眩：病症名，因风邪、风痰所致的眩晕。

### 97. Niu ［牛, cattle, Bovidae］

As a livestock, it is relied on as agricultural labour and it is seldom killed. If it dies naturally, its blood vessels have been expired and its bone marrow has been exhausted, and then its meat is inedible. Huangniu ［黄牛, cattle, Bos Taurus］ can cause toxic side effects and some diseases. Heiniu ［黑牛, water buffalo, Bubalus］, whose urine and feces can be used as medicine, is especially inedible.

Its head and hoofs can be used to treat the wind heat[1], but they are inedible for the people suffering from deficiency cold.

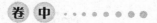

Its liver can be used to treat dysentery. And taking it can treat emaciation if boiled with vinegar.

Its tripe boiled with vinegar can be used to treat the consumptive thirst and wind dizziness[2], and tonify the five zang-organs.

Its kidney is mainly used to tonify kidneys.

Its bone marrow is used to quiet the five zang-organs, calm the triple energizer and warm the middle. Long-term taking of it will prolong life. It should be taken with liquor. The decoction of the bone marrow of Heiniu〔黑牛,water buffalo, Bubalus〕in equal proportion with Dihuangzhi〔地黄汁, fresh rehmannia juice, Rehmanniae Radicis Recentis Succus〕and honey can be used to treat emaciation. But be cautious of purposefully using decocted cattle fat instead.

The decoction of its dung is mainly used to treat cholera, particularly the dung of Heiniu〔黑牛, water buffalo, Bubalus〕is recommended as the most effective one. If a child is crying at night, take a piece of dried dung the size of the palm and place it under the bed mat without telling the mother, then the child and the mother will get better.

Women take the thick soup of its nose on an empty stomach, which can help them produce milk. A large amount of milk will come in two or three days. It is quite effective for those middle-aged and strong women.

It is inedible if it is killed, let alone it dies naturally. Take 3 Jin of beef and cut it into pieces to feed the fierce horse that tends to escape from the manger and bite people, the horse will become tame and gentle after fed twice. After fed three or five times, the horse will become weak, stupid and unable to ride. Don't take beef in the twelfth lunar month because it can hurt people's spirit.

【Notes】

〔1〕wind heat: A disease caused by the invasion of pathogenic factors of wind and heat.

〔2〕wind dizziness: A dizziness disease caused by wind evil or wind phlegm.

## 98. 牛 乳 寒

（一）患热风人宜服之。患冷气人不宜服之。

（二）乌牛乳酪：寒。主热毒，止渴，除胸中热。

## 98．Niuru［牛乳，cow's milk，Bovis Lac］*cold*

It is good for those suffering from the heat wind, but not suitable for those suffering from cold qi.

The cheese of Heiniu［黑牛，water buffalo，Bubalus］is cold in property, and mainly used to resolve the heat toxin, relieve thirst and eliminate the heat evil in the chest.

## 99．羊

（一）角：主惊邪，明目，辟鬼，安心益气。烧角作灰，治鬼气并漏下恶血。

（二）羊肉：温。主风眩瘦病，小儿惊痫，丈夫五劳七伤[1]，藏气虚寒。河西[2]羊最佳，河东[3]羊亦好。纵驱至南方，筋力自劳损，安能补益人？

（三）羊肉：妊娠人勿多食。患天行及疟人食，令发热困重致死。

（四）头肉：平。主缓中，汗出虚劳，安心止惊。宿有冷病人勿多食。主热风眩，疫疾[4]，小儿痫，兼补胃虚损及丈夫五劳骨热[5]。热病后宜食羊头肉。

（五）肚：主补胃病虚损，小便数，止虚汗。以肥肚作羹食，三五度瘥。

（六）肝：性冷[6]。治肝风虚热[6]，目赤暗痛，热病后失明者，以青羊肝或子肝薄切，水浸敷之，极效。生子肝吞之尤妙。主目失明，取羖羊肝一斤，去脂膜薄切，以未著水新瓦盆一口，揩令净，铺肝于盆中，置于炭火上煿，令脂汁尽。候极干，取决明子半升，蓼子一合，炒令香为末，和肝杵之为末。以白蜜浆下方寸匕。食后服之，日三，加至三匕止，不过二剂，目极明。一年服之妙，夜见文字并诸物。

（七）其羖羊，即骨历羊是也。常患眼痛涩，不能视物，及看日光并灯火光不得者，取熟羊头眼睛中白珠子二枚，于细石上和枣汁研之，取如小麻子大，安眼睛上，仰卧。日二夜二，不过三四度瘥。

（八）羊心：补心肺，从三月至五月，其中有虫如马尾毛，长二三寸已来。须割去之，不去令人痫。

（九）羊毛：醋煮裹脚，治转筋。

（十）又，取皮去毛煮羹，补虚劳。煮作臛食之，去一切风，治脚中虚风[7]。

（十一）羊骨：热。主治虚劳，患宿热[8]人勿食。

（十二）髓：酒服之，补血。主女人风血虚闷。

（十三）头中髓：发风。若和酒服，则迷人心，便成中风也。

（十四）羊屎：黑人毛发。主箭镞不出。粪和雁膏敷毛发落，三宿生。

（十五）白羊黑头者，勿食之。令人患肠痈[9]。一角羊不可食。六月勿食羊，伤神。

（十六）谨按：南方羊都不与盐食之，多在山中吃野草，或食毒草。若北羊，一二年间亦不可食，食必病生尔。为其来南地食毒草故也。若南地人食之，即不忧也。今将北羊于南地养三年之后，犹亦不中食，何况于南羊能堪食乎？盖土地各然也。

【注释】

[1] 五劳七伤："五劳"是指心、肝、脾、肺、肾五脏劳损；"七伤"是指喜、怒、悲、忧、恐、惊、思七情伤害。此处泛指各种虚损证。

[2] 河西：古地名，约今甘肃一带，因位于黄河以西，故称为"河西"。

[3] 河东：古地名，古代指山西西南部，因在黄河以东，故称为"河东"。

[4] 疫疾：流行的传染病。另外，根据第二条这里似乎应该是瘦疾。

[5] 骨热：病症名，湿气侵入骨头引起，其特点是骨有炎症，全身发热。主要临床表现为疼痛。

[6] 虚热：病症名，多因内伤劳损所致。

[7] 脚中虚风：腿脚因为受虚风侵袭而软弱无力；虚风指非当令季节所来的风，失时之风，如春季刮的西风、夏季刮的北风等。

[8] 宿热：病症名，脏腑之气与热相搏引起的疾病。

[9] 肠痈：病症名，痈疽之发肠部者，多由湿热、气滞、血瘀等留注肠中，气血郁阻所致。多见于西医学所说急性阑尾炎、阑尾周围脓肿等。

## 99. Yang［羊，goat，Merycoidodon Gracilis］

Its horn is mainly used to treat diseases caused by fright, improve vision, repel non-auspicious pathogenic factors like ghost, quiet the heart and replenish qi. Its burnt ash can be used to eliminate the ghost qi（pathogenic factors）and treat the vaginal discharge of blood stasis.

Mutton, warm in property, is mainly used to treat the wind dizziness, emaciation, fright epilepsy in children, men's five kinds of overstrain and seven kinds of damage[1], and deficiency-cold of viscera. The goat in Hexi[2] is the best, and the one in Hedong[3] is next only to it. However, if the goat is driven to the south, its sinews and bones will be strained due to the long-distance trudge. How can it tonify people?

Pregnant women should not eat mutton excessively. If those who suffer from epidemics or malaria take mutton, the heat evil will become more severe and stays still in their bodies, and could make them dead.

The mutton of its head, mild in property, is mainly used to harmonize the middle energizer, treat the vacuity-taxation sweating, quiet the heart and relieve fright. Those who suffered from deficiency cold should not take much. It is mainly used to treat heat wind dizziness, epidemic diseases[4] and epilepsy in children, as well as tonify the stomach vacuity detriment and treat men's five kinds of overstrain and heat in the bones[5]. It is suitable for a man suffering from heat disease to take it.

Its tripe is mainly to tonify the stomach vacuity detriment, treat the frequent micturition and cease the deficiency sweating. People suffering from the diseases mentioned above can be cured after taking three or five times of thick soup made by fat tripe.

Its liver, cold in property, can be used to treat the liver wind vacuity heat[6] and red eyes with pain and blurred vision. The water-soaked slices of liver of indigo goats and lambs are very effective in treating the blindness caused by heat disease when applying to eyes, and eating raw lambs' livers is especially effective. To treat blindness, take 1 Jin of the liver of black male goats, remove fat and fascia and slice it, then take a new clay pot never touched by water and clean it, spread the liver slices in the bottom of pot, and bake the pot with charcoal fire until the fat in the livers is gone completely and the liver becomes very dry and crisp.

Take half a Sheng of Juemingzi [决明子, fetid cassia, Cassiae Semen] and 1 Ge of Liaozicao [蓼子草, slender bearded smartweed, Polygoni Gracilis Herba et Radix], stir-fry them until smelling fragrant, grind them into powder, and pestle the powder and the liver slices into a new powder. Take 1 Fangcunbi (square-cun-spoon) of the powder with honey three times a day after meal. Gradually increase the amount of each dose until it is up to a maximum of 3 Fangcunbi (square-cun-spoon). After two more doses, the patient will have a very clear vision. It is

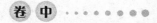

better to take it for one year, and by then the patient will read and see at night.

The black male goat is also called Guli goat (骨历羊). If suffering from dry and sore eyes, difficult to see clearly, and daring not see the sun and the lights, take two eye whites from the cooked head of the black male goat, and grind them with the juice of Dazao〔大枣, jujube, Jujubae Fructus〕on a fine stone, apply as much as the amount in size of a cannabis fruit to the eyeball and then lie on the back, apply it twice in the day and twice at night, the eyes will be cured in three or four days.

Its heart can be used to tonify the heart and the lung. From the third lunar month to the fifth lunar month, there is a kind of worms in the goat's heart which is like horsetail hair and is about 2 or 3 Cun long. The worms should be eliminated or they will cause dysentery.

Its wool, if boiled with vinegar, can be used to treat cramp by wrapping it around the feet.

Its dehaired skin, boiled into thick soup, can tonify the vacuity taxation. Taking the soup can eliminate all wind evils and treat the weak legs and feet due to the invasion of deficiency wind[7].

Its bones, hot in property, are mainly used to treat deficiency due to overstrain. Those who suffered from heat-qi disease[8] should not take it.

Its bone marrow can tonify the blood when taken with liquor. It is mainly used to treat the women's vexation and oppression caused by blood vacuity.

Its brain marrow can cause the wind evil disease. If taken with liquor, it will confuse people's mind which can cause a stroke.

Its manure can black hair and treat the disease caused by arrow head deep in the flesh. Mix the manure with the fat of Yan〔雁, swan goose, Anser Cygnoides〕and apply them to head where the hair is shed, hair will grow out in three nights.

The white goat with a black head is inedible because it will cause the intestinal welling-abscess[9]. The single-horn one is inedible either. Don't take it in the sixth lunar month because it can hurt people's spirit.

The following is supplemented by Zhang Ding: People don't feed the salty food to goat in the south. The southern one is usually fed on wild grass in the mountains and sometimes eat the toxic grass. Even if from the north it is inedible after it lives in the south for one or two years. People will definitely get sick if they eat it because it will eat the toxic grass after coming to the south. However, it is all right for the southern locals. Even the northern one becomes inedible after it lives in the south for three years. How can the original southern one be edible? It lies in the reason that the land conditions are different.

【Notes】

[1] five kinds of overstrain and seven kinds of damage: Generally the five kinds of overstrain refer to the overstrain of five organs of heart, liver, spleen, lungs and kidneys; the seven kinds of damage refer to the damage caused by the seven affects of delight, anger, sadness, sorrow, fear, shock and missing. Here they refer to the diseases caused by the vacuity detriment.

[2] Hexi: Also known as Hexi Corridor, it refers to the area of west of the Yellow River, and it is mainly in Gansu Province today.

[3] Hedong: It refers to the area of east of the Yellow River, and it is mainly in the southwest of Shanxi Province today.

[4] epidemic diseases: According to the second clause of the original text, here it should probably be "emanciation" instead of "epidemic disease". Chinese character "疫"(epidemic disease) is similar to the character "瘦"(emaciation) in writing.

[5] heat in the bones: A disease, which is caused by the invasion of damp into the bones, characterized by a series of inflammatory reactions in the bones and fever throughout the body. Usually the main clinical manifestation is featured by pain.

[6] liver wind vacuity heat: A disease caused by the invasion of wind into the liver, the internal injuries and overstrain.

[7] deficiency wind: The wind that is not in season. For example, the west wind in spring or the north wind in summer.

[8] heat-qi disease: A disease caused by the organ qi and heat contending with each other.

[9] intestinal welling-abscess: A disease, referring to the intestinal carbuncle caused by damp heat, qi stagnation, blood stasis, etc. in the intestines which cause qi and blood obstruction. It is similar to acute appendicitis, abscess around the appendix, etc. in Western medicine.

# 100. 羊 乳

（一）补肺肾气[1]，和小肠。亦主消渴，治虚劳，益精气。合脂作羹食，补肾虚。
（二）羊乳治卒心痛，可温服之。
（三）亦主女子与男子中风。蚰蜒[2]入耳，以羊乳灌耳中即成水。
（四）又，主小儿口中烂疮，取羖羊生乳，含五六日瘥。

**【注释】**

［1］肺肾气：肺气为肺的生理功能；肾气为肾脏的功能活动。

［2］蚰蜒：节肢动物，像蜈蚣而略小，体色黄褐。

## 100. Yangru［羊乳，goat's milk，Caprae seu Ovis Lac］

It can tonify the lung-kidney qi[1] and harmonize the small intestines. It can also treat the consumptive thirst and deficiency due to overstrain, and replenish the essential qi. The thick soap made with it and Yangzhi［羊脂, goat's fat, Caprae seu Ovis Adeps］can treat the kidney deficiency.

Taking it warm can treat the sudden pain in the heart.

It can treat the stroke of both male and female. If a scutiger[2] in the ear, drop it into the ear, the scutiger then will turn into water.

It can also treat the severe sores in the mouth of children. Hold the fresh milk of black goats in the mouth and the sores will be cured in five or six days.

**【Notes】**

［1］lung-kidney qi: The lung qi is the physiological function of the lung and the kidney qi is the functional activity of the kidney.

［2］scutiger: A kind of arthropod which has a yellow body and fifteen pairs of slender legs. It is similar to a centipede but slightly smaller.

## 101. 酥 寒

（一）除胸中热，补五藏，利肠胃。
（二）水牛酥功同，寒，与羊酪同功。羊酥真者胜牛酥。

### 101. Su〔酥, butter, Bovis seu Ovis Butyrum〕*cold*

It can eliminate the heat in the chest, tonify the five zang-organs and promote function of the stomach and intestines.

Shuiniusu〔水牛酥, water buffalo's butter, Bubali Butyrum〕, cold in property, has the same effects as Yangsu〔羊酥, goat's butter, Caprae seu Ovis Byturum〕. The authentic Yangsu〔羊酥, goat's butter, Caprae seu Ovis Byturum〕is better than Niusu〔牛酥, cow's milk butter, Bovis Butyrum〕.

### 102. 酪[1] 寒

主热毒,止渴,除胃中热。患冷人勿食羊乳酪。
【注释】
[1] 酪:用牛、马、羊、骆驼等动物的乳汁炼制而成的半凝固或凝固的乳制品。

### 102. Lao〔酪, cheese[1], Ceseus〕*cold*

It is mainly used to resolve the heat toxin, relieve thirst and eliminate the heat evil in the stomach. Those suffering from the deficiency cold should not eat it.
【Note】
[1] cheese:A kind of semi-solidified or solidified dairy food made from the milk of cow, mare, goat or camel.

### 103. 醍 醐[1] 平

主风邪,通润骨髓。性冷利,乃酥之本精液也。
【注释】
[1] 醍醐:从酥酪中提制出的油。

### 103. Tihu〔醍醐, butter oil[1], Bovis Butyri Oleum〕*mild*

It is mainly used to treat the diseases caused by the wind evil, and enrich and moisten the bone marrow. Cold in property and smooth in taste, it is the essence of butter.

【Note】

[1] butter oil: A kind of oil extracted from butter or cheese.

# 104. 乳　腐[1]

微寒。润五藏,利大小便,益十二经脉[2]。微动气。细切如豆,面拌,醋浆水[3]煮二十余沸,治赤白痢。小儿患,服之弥佳。

【注释】

[1] 乳腐:为牛乳等乳类的加工制成品,也称为"乳饼",具有润肠通便、健脾止痢之功效。

[2] 十二经脉:经络系统的主体,具有表里经脉相合、与相应脏腑络属的主要特征,包括手三阴经(手太阴肺经、手厥阴心包经、手少阴心经)、手三阳经(手阳明大肠经、手少阳三焦经、手太阳小肠经)、足三阳经(足阳明胃经、足少阳胆经、足太阳膀胱经)、足三阴经(足太阴脾经、足厥阴肝经、足少阴肾经),也称为"正经"。

[3] 醋浆水:也称为"浆水",中药材名。本品为用粟米加工、经发酵而成的白色浆液。

# 104. Rufu [乳腐, curd[1], Lac Pressum]

Slightly cold in property, it can be used to enrich and moisten the five zang-organs, disinhibit urination and defecation and replenish the twelve channels[2]. It can slightly stir qi. It can be used to treat the red and white dysentery after finely cut into pea-sized pieces, mixed with flour and boiled in Cujiangshui [醋浆水, sour millet water[3], Setariae Praeparatum Liquidum] until the water boils more than 20 times. It is very effective in treating the infantile diseases.

【Notes】

[1] curd: It is also called milk cake and is a processed product made from milk, having the effect of moistening the intestine, disinhibiting defecation, fortifying the spleen and checking dysentery.

[2] twelve channels: A collective term for the three yin meridians and three yang meridians of each hand and foot. It is also called twelve regular meridians. They are characterized by corresponding to those of the zang-fu organs. They are shou san yin jing (three yin channels of the hand), including shou tai yin fei jing (hand greater yin lung channel; LU), shou jue yin xin bao jing (hand reverting yin pericardium channel; PC), shou shao yin xin jing (hand lesser yin heart channel; HT); shou san yang jing (three yang channels of the hand), including shou yang ming da chang jing (hand yang brightness large intestine channel; LI), shou shao yang san jiao jing (hand lesser yang triple energizer channel; TB), shou tai yang xiao chang jing (hand greater yang small intestine channel; SI); zu san yang jing (three yang channels of the foot) including zu yang ming wei jing (foot yang brightness stomach channel; ST), zu shao yang dan jing (foot lesser yang gallbladder channel; GB), zu tai yang pang guang jing (foot greater yang bladder channel; BL); zu san yin jing (foot greater yin spleen channel; SP), zu jue yin gan jing (foot reverting yin liver channel; LV), zu shao yin shen jing (foot lesser yin kidney channel; KI).

[3] sour millet water: A kind of medicinal material. It is also called millet water. It is made from millet and becomes the white slurry after fermentation.

# 105. 马

（一）白马黑头，食令人癫。白马自死，食之害人。

（二）肉：冷，有小毒。主肠中热，除下气[1]，长筋骨。

（三）不与仓米同食，必卒得恶，十有九死。不与姜同食，生气嗽。其肉多著浸洗方煮，得烂熟兼去血尽，始可煮食。肥者亦然，不尔毒不出。

（四）又，食诸马肉心闷，饮清酒[2]即解，浊酒[3]即加。

（五）赤马蹄：主辟温疟[4]。

（六）悬蹄[5]：主惊痫。

（七）又，恶刺疮，取黑（駮）马尿热渍，当（虫出）愈。数数洗之。

（八）白秃疮，以駮马不乏者尿，数数暖洗之十遍，瘥。

（九）患丁肿[6]，中风疼痛者，炒驴马粪，熨疮满五十遍，极效。患杖疮[7]并打损疮，中风疼痛者，炒马驴湿粪，分取半，替换热熨之。冷则易之，日五十遍[8],极效。

（十）男子患,未可及,新瘥后,合阴阳,垂至死,取白马粪五升,绞取汁,好器中盛停一宿,一服三合,日夜二服。

（十一）又,小儿患头疮[9],烧马骨作灰,和醋敷。亦治身上疮。

（十二）又,白马脂五两,封疮上。稍稍封之,白秃者发即生。

（十三）又,马汗入人疮,毒气攻作脓,心懑欲绝者,烧粟杆草作灰,浓淋作浓灰汁,热煮,蘸疮于灰汁中,须臾白沫出尽即瘥。白沫者,是毒气也。此方岭南新有人曾得力。

（十四）凡生马血入人肉中,多只三两日便肿,连心则死。有人剥马,被骨伤手指,血入肉中,一夜致死。

（十五）又,臆胘,次胅胘也。蹄无夜眼[10]者勿食。又黑脊而斑不可食。患疮疥人切不得食,加增难瘥。

（十六）赤马皮临产铺之,令产母坐上催生。

（十七）白马茎:益丈夫阴气,阴干者末,和苁蓉蜜丸,空腹酒下四十丸,日再,百日见效。

（十八）（马心）:患痢人不得食。

**【注释】**

［1］下气:指肠胃郁结而形成的气。

［2］［3］浊酒,清酒:古人主要用黍和稻酿酒,称为“黍酒”,就是我们今天所说的黄酒。浊酒就是没有经过过滤的黍酒,因为有酒渣在里面;而清酒就是滤去渣滓的酒。

［4］温疟:夏季感受暑热而发的一种疟疾,临床表现有先热后寒、热重寒轻、汗或多或少、口渴喜凉饮、舌红等症状。

［5］悬蹄:马蹄后部上方不落地的小蹄。

［6］丁肿:丁疮。

［7］杖疮:受杖刑后的创伤。

［8］日五十遍:有说应为满五十遍。

［9］头疮:现代医学称之为多发性头部毛囊炎,是临床常见的皮肤病。

［10］夜眼:马膝上所生皮肤角质块。

### 105. Ma [马, horse, Equus Caballus]

A white Ma [马, horse, Equus Caballus] with a black head is inedible because it will cause epilepsy. It is harmful to eat the white one that dies naturally.

Its meat, cold and slightly toxic in property, is mainly used to treat the heat evil in the intestines, eliminate lower body qi[1] and strengthen the sinews and bones.

Don't eat its meat with the old rice, otherwise it will definitely cause the severe illnesses ten to one resulting in death. Don't eat the meat with Shengjiang [生姜, fresh ginger, Zingiberis Rhizoma Recens] because it will cause cough. Before eating its meat, soak and wash it several times and cook it thoroughly to make the blood completely gone. The fat meat should be also processed like that, otherwise the toxin inside will not be eliminated.

Eating its meat may cause the oppression in the heart, which can be resolved by drinking some clear liquor[2] but drinking turbid liquor[3] will make the symptom more severe.

The hoof of red Ma [马, horse, Equus Caballus] is mainly used to repel the warm malaria[4].

Its suspended hoof[5] is mainly used to treat the fright epilepsy.

The urine of the black Ma [马, horse, Equus Caballus] (or the one with blue and white hair) can be used to treat the sore caused by the piecing of the toxic thorn. Soak the sore surface in the hot urine to force the worms out and the sore will be healed. It is necessary to wash the sore surface several times.

The urine of the one which has blue and white hair and seldom feels tired can be used to treat the bald scalp sore. Use the hot urine to wash the sore surface more than ten times and the sore will be healed.

Its dung can be used to treat the clove sore[6] and the pain caused by the wind evil. Stir-fry the dung, wrap it in gauze and apply it to the sore surface fifty times while it is hot. It is extremely effective. To treat the rod sore[7], the sore caused by the traumatic injury and pain caused by the wind evil, stir-fry the wet dung of Ma [马, horse, Equus Caballus] and Lü [驴, donkey, Equus Asinus], divide it into two halves, wrap it in gauze and apply it to the sore surface in turn while it is hot. Switch to the hot one when the wrapped dung is cool. Apply it to the surface fifty times a day[8]. It is extremely effective.

A man is dying due to the recurrence of his old disease caused by the sexsual activities when he is not recovered or just recovered from his illness. To treat the man take 5 Sheng of dung of white Ma [马, horse, Equus Caballus], wring out the juice and put the juice in a clean container for one night. The man should drink the juice 3 Ge at a time and drink it twice every day and night.

To treat a child who suffers from the head sore[9], burn its bones to ash and apply the ash to the sore with vinegar. It can also be used to treat the sore in the body.

To treat the patient who suffers from the bald scalp sore, take 5 Liang of fat of the white Ma [马, horse, Equus Caballus] and apply a thin layer of it to the sore surface. The hair will grow up soon.

If its sweat goes into the sore of a patient, the invasion of the toxic qi will cause suppuration, which makes the patient dying due to the vexation and oppression in the heart and chest. To treat the patient, burn the millet rod to ash, drench the ash to get thick ash juice, boil the juice and soak the sore surface in the juice. Some white foam will come out right away and the patient will be cured when there is no foam coming out. The white foam is toxic qi. It was effective in treating the patient in Lingnan not long ago.

If its fresh blood goes into the flesh of a person, the flesh will swell up in two or three days at most. The person will die if the swelling affects the heart. A man died overnight when he peeled a Ma [马, horse, Equus Caballus] and was hurt by its bones which made its blood go into his flesh.

People suffering from sores and scabies should not eat the fat in its chest and belly because it will make the disease more severe and difficult to be cured. The one without Yeyan[10] on its hooves or the one with spots on its black back is inedible.

A woman in labor can sit on a hide of a red one which can hasten the delivery.

The penis of the white Ma [马, horse, Equus Caballus] can be used to improve men's sexual ability. Dry the penis in the shade, grind it into powder, make it into pills with Congrong [苁蓉, cistanche, Cistanches Herba] and take forty pills with liquor on an empty stomach twice a day. It will be effective after 100 days of taking.

People who suffer from dysentery should not eat its heart.

【Notes】

［1］lower body qi：It refers to the qi caused by the gastrointestinal stagnation.

［2］［3］clear liquor and turbid liquor：The ancients mainly used millet and rice to make liquor which was called Shujiu, actually the yellow rice liquor today. The turbid liquor is the unfiltered liquor with lees in it and the clear liquor is the filtered liquor.

［4］warm malaria：A malaria caused by heat in summer. The clinical manifestations include cold after hot, severe hot and less severe cold, much or little sweat, thirst, desiring for cold drink, red tongue, etc.

［5］suspended hoof：The small hoof on the above part of the back of the horse hoof, which does not touch the ground.

［6］clove sore：It is also called deep-rooted boil.

［7］rod sore：The wounds caused by the punishment of flogging.

［8］fifty times a day：In another book it is said that there are altogether fifty times.

［9］head sore：It is called multiple head folliculitis in modern medicine. It is a common clinical skin disease.

［10］Yeyan：The horny block in the horse's lap.

# 106. 黄明胶[1]（白胶）

（一）敷肿四边,中心留一孔子,其肿即头自开也。

（二）治咳嗽不瘥者,黄明胶炙令半焦为末,每服一钱匕,人参末二钱匕,用薄豉汤一钱八分[2],葱少许,入铫子[3]煎一两沸后,倾入盏,遇咳嗽时呷三五口后,依前温暖,却准前咳嗽时吃之也。

（三）又,止吐血,咯血,黄明胶一两,切作小片子,炙令黄;新绵一两,烧作灰细研,每服一钱匕,新米饮调下,不计年岁深远并宜,食后卧时服。

【注释】

［1］黄明胶:唐代时期的黄明胶就是白胶,也就是鹿角胶。宋代以后的黄明胶指的是用牛皮熬制而成的胶。

［2］一钱八分:参考其他文章,"钱"应为"盏","八分"为多余的文字。因

此,这里原文应为"用薄豉汤一盏"。盏,又称"器皿",是指盛装液体的日常器具,材质通常为陶瓷、木、竹、金属等。常用物品如茶盏、油盏、灯盏。

[3] 铫子:铫子就是煎药或烧水用的器具,形状像比较高的壶,口大有盖,旁边有柄,用沙土或金属制成。

## 106. Huangmingjiao (Baijiao)[1][黄明胶(白胶),
### deerhorn glue, Cervi Cornus Gelatinum]

Apply it to the skin around the toxin swelling instead of the central part, where the toxin swelling will form a pus head which will erupt itself.

To treat the cough lasting a long time, broil it until it is half-charred and grind it into powder. Put 1 Qianbi of the powder, 2 Qianbi of Renshen [人参, ginseng, Ginseng Radix] powder, 1 Zhan[2] of the thin decoction of Douchi [豆豉, fermented soybean, Sojae Semen Fermentatum] and a little Cong [葱, scallion, Allii Fistulosi Herba] into a Diaozi[3] and boil them for a couple of times. Then pour the liquid into cup and sip a little while coughing. Reheat the liquid according to the previous method and drink it when feeling like coughing.

To treat the spitting blood or hemoptysis, cut 1 Liang of it into small slices and broil it until it turns yellow. Burn 1 Liang of new Mian [绵, silk floss, Bombycis Lana] to ash. Grind the broiled slices and the ash into fine powder. Drink 1 Qianbi of the powder with the soup cooked by new rice. It is suitable for a patient to drink it no matter how long the patient has been suffering from the disease. The patient should drink it after supper before going to bed.

**[Notes]**

[1] Huangming jiao (Baijiao): In the Tang Dynasty, it was also called Baijiao (白胶), referring to deerhorn glue. After the Song Dynasty it referred to the glue made from cow hide.

[2] 1 Zhan: Referring to other articles, "钱" (Qian) of the original text should be "盏"(Zhan) and "八分" (8 Fen) are unnecessary characters and should be omitted.

[3] Diaozi: A kind of utensil used for decocting herbal medicine or boiling water. It is similar to a tall pot with a large mouth and a lid. It has a handle and is made of sand soil or metal.

# 107. 犬（狗）

（一）牡狗阴茎：补髓。

（二）犬肉：益阳事，补血脉，厚肠胃，实下焦，填精髓。不可炙食，恐成消渴。但和五味煮，空腹食之。不与蒜同食，必顿损人。若去血则力少，不益人。瘦者多是病，不堪食。比来去血食之，却不益人也。肥者血亦香美，即何要去血？去血之后，都无效矣。

（三）肉：温。主五藏，补七伤五劳，填骨髓，大补益气力。空腹食之。黄色牡者上，白、黑色者次。女人妊娠勿食。

（四）胆：去肠中脓水[1]。

（五）又，上伏日[2]采胆，以酒调服之。明目，去眼中脓水。

（六）又，白犬胆和通草、桂为丸服，令人隐形[3]。青犬尤妙。

（七）又，主恶疮痂痒，以胆汁敷之止。胆敷恶疮，能破血。有中伤因损者，热酒调半个服，瘀血尽下。

（八）又，犬伤人，杵生杏仁封之瘥。

（九）犬自死，舌不出者，食之害人。九月勿食犬肉，伤神。

【注释】

[1] 肠中脓水：根据原文第五条，这里似乎应该是"去眼中脓水"。

[2] 上伏日：初伏。三伏分为初伏、中伏、末伏。

[3] 隐形：这是一种古人的迷信，肯定没有科学道理，不可能是真的。

## 107. Quan（Gou）［犬（狗），dog，Canis Lupus Familiaris］

The penis of the male Gou［狗，dog，Canis lupus familiaris］can be used to replenish the essence and marrow.

Its meat can be used to improve men's sexual ability, tonify the blood vessels, strengthen the function of the stomach and intestines, and enrich the lower energizer and the essence and marrow. Don't eat the broiled meat for fear of causing the consumptive thirst. Its meat should be cooked with the ordinary cooking seasonings and eaten on an empty stomach. Don't eat the meat with garlic, or health would be damaged in a moment. If the blood in the meat is gone, the meat will not benefit people. The thin Gou〔狗, dog, Canis Lupus Familiaris〕 is inedible for it is often getting ill. In the past, people would remove the blood before eating its meat. In fact, it didn't benefit people. Why is it necessary to remove the blood since the blood of the fat one is also delicious? If the blood in the meat is gone, the meat will not be effective.

Its meat, warm in property, is mainly used to tonify the five zang-organs, treat men's five kinds of overstrain and seven kinds of damage, enrich the bone marrow and greatly replenish qi and energy. It should be eaten on an empty stomach. The meat of the yellow male one is the best and the meat of the white or black one is next only to it. Pregnant women shouldn't eat the meat.

Its gall can be used to eliminate the pus in the intestines[1].

Taking the gall collected during Chufu[2] with liquor can improve vision and eliminate the pus in the eyes.

Taking the pills made of the gall of the white Gou〔狗, dog, Canis Lupus Familiaris〕 with Tongcao〔通草, rice-paper plant pith, Tetrapanacis Medulla〕 and Rougui〔肉桂, cinnamon bark, Cinnamomi Cortex〕 has the function of physical invisibility[3]. The gall of the indigo one has a better effect.

The bile is mainly used to treat the itching from the crusting of the severe sore. Apply it to the crust, the itching will be gone, and to the severe sore, the blood stasis will be gone as well. If injured, take the bile of half a gall with hot liquor to completely eliminate the blood stasis.

If bitten by a Gou〔狗, dog, Canis Lupus Familiaris〕, apply the pestled raw Xingren〔杏仁, apricot kernel, Armeniacae Semen〕 to the wound.

It is harmful to eat the dog without tongue sticking out after dying naturally. Don't eat its meat in the ninth lunar month because it can hurt people's spirit.

【Notes】

〔1〕 pus in the intestines: According to the fifth clause of the original text, here it should probably be "eyes" instead of "intestines". Chinese character "肠" (intestines) is similar to the character "眼" (eyes) in writing.

〔2〕 Chufu: In Chinese culture, the hot summer is divided into three periods, Chufu, Zhongfu and Mofu.

〔3〕 function of physical invisibility: It was a superstitious belief in ancient China, which of course is not scientific and can't be true.

# 108. 兔

（一）肝：主明目，和决明子作丸服之。

（二）又，主丹石人上冲眼暗不见物，可生食之，一如服羊子肝法。

（三）兔头骨并同肉：味酸。

（四）谨按：八月至十月，其肉酒炙[1]吃，与丹石人甚相宜。注：以性冷故也[2]。大都绝人血脉，损房事，令人痿黄。

（五）肉：不宜与姜、橘同食之，令人卒患心痛，不可治也。

（六）又，兔死而眼合者，食之杀人。二月食之伤神。

（七）又，兔与生姜同食，成霍乱。

【注释】

[1] 酒炙：中药的一种炮制方法。将净药材加酒拌匀，闷透，置锅内，用文火炒至规定程度时，取出放凉。

[2] 此注原注者不明。

## 108. Tu［兔，rabbit，Oryctolagus Cuniculus］

Its liver is mainly used to improve vision. Make the liver into pills with Juemingzi［决明子，fetid cassia，Cassiae Semen］and take them.

Its liver can also be mainly used to treat the person who has dim vision and can't see things clearly because of the upsurge of the toxin in the Danshi he takes. Take the raw liver just like taking the raw lamb's liver.

Its skull and meat are sour in taste.

The following is supplemented by Zhang Ding: The person who takes Danshi is suitable to eat its meat mix-fried with liquor[1] between the eighth lunar month and the tenth lunar month. Note: This is because its meat is cold in property[2]. Its meat can often make people's blood vessels expired, damage their sexual ability and make them have yellow facial complexion.

It is unsuitable to eat its meat with Shengjiang［生姜，fresh ginger，Zingiberis Rhizoma Recens］and Ju［橘，tangerine，Citrus Reticulata］because it will cause the sudden pain in the heart, which is incurable.

It is lethal to eat one that dies with its eyes closed. Eating its meat in the second lunar month can hurt people's spirit.

Eating the meat with Shengjiang〔生姜, fresh ginger, Zingiberis Rhizoma Recens〕can cause cholera.

【Notes】

〔1〕mix-fried with liquor: A processing method of Chinese medicinals. It is to mix evenly the clean medicinal materials with liquor, cover them tightly, put them in a pot, stir-fry them over a low flame to a prescribed degree and take them out for cooling.

〔2〕The author of this note is unknown.

# 109. 猪(豚)

(一) 肉:味苦,微寒。压丹石,疗热闭血脉。虚人动风,不可久食。令人少子精,发宿疹。主疗人肾虚。肉发痰,若患疟疾人切忌食,必再发。

(二) 肾:主人肾虚,不可久食。

(三) 江猪:平。肉酸。多食令人体重。今捕人作脯,多皆不识。但食,少有腥气。

(四) 又,舌:和五味煮取汁饮,能健脾,补不足之气,令人能食。

(五) 大猪头:主补虚,乏气力,去惊痫、五痔,下丹石。

(六) 又,肠:主虚渴[1],小便数,补下焦虚竭[2]。

(七) 东行母猪粪一升,宿浸,去滓顿服,治毒黄热病。

(八) 肚:主暴痢虚弱。

【注释】

〔1〕虚渴:分为阳虚口渴和阴虚口渴。阳虚口渴是因为阳气虚弱不能蒸腾津液上承所导致,而阴虚口渴是因为阴虚津液不足所导致。

〔2〕下焦虚竭:下焦脏器功能的虚损衰竭。

## 109. Zhu (Tun)〔猪(豚), pig (finless porpoise), Sus Scrofa Domestica (Neophocaena Asiaeorientalis)〕

Zhurou〔猪肉, pork, Suis Caro〕, bitter in taste and slightly cold in property, can resolve the toxin of Danshi and treat the obstructed blood vessels caused by the heat evil. It will cause wind qi to a person in weak heath if he eats it, so he shouldn't have a long-term eating of it. Eating it can make a man have fewer sperms and cause the recurrence of his old diseases. It is mainly used to treat the kidney deficiency. It can cause the abundant phlegm. Those suffering from malaria are especially forbidden to eat it, otherwise there will be definitely the recurrence of the disease.

The kidney of Zhu〔猪, pig, Sus Scrofa Domestica〕is mainly used to treat the kidney deficiency, but people shouldn't have a long-term eating of it.

The meat of Jiangzhu〔江猪, finless porpoise, Neophocaena Asiaeorientalis〕is sour in taste and mild in property. Eating it excessively will make people gain weight. Now hunters make it into dried meat and few people can recognize it. They just eat it and it tastes slightly fishy.

Cook the tongue of Zhu〔猪, pig, Sus Scrofa Domestica〕with the ordinary cooking seasonings to make soup. Drinking the soup can fortify the spleen, supplement the insufficient qi and make people eat more.

The head of big Zhu〔猪, pig, Sus Scrofa Domestica〕is mainly used to supplement deficiency, treat the lack of strength, fright epilepsy and five kinds of hemorrhoids, and resolve the toxin of Danshi.

The intestines of Zhu〔猪, pig, Sus Scrofa Domestica〕is mainly used to treat the deficiency thirst[1] and urinary frequency, and tonify the lower energizer exhaustion[2].

Take 1 Sheng of manure of the sow that goes east, soak it in water for one night, filter it and take it at a time. It can cure the jaundice and heat disease caused by heat evil.

The tripe of Zhu〔猪, pig, Sus Scrofa Domestica〕is mainly used to treat the weakness caused by acute dysentery.

**【Notes】**

〔1〕deficiency thirst: It includes yang deficiency thirst and yin deficiency thirst. Yang deficiency thirst is caused by yang qi deficiency which can't transpire the fluids to make it bear upward. Yin deficiency thirst is caused by yin qi deficiency which leads to fluids deficiency.

[2] lower energizer exhaustion: It means the function of the lower energizer organs exhausts.

# 110. 驴

（一）肉：主风狂，忧愁不乐，能安心气。

（二）又，头：焊去毛，煮汁以渍曲酿酒，去大风。

（三）又，生脂和生椒熟捣，绵裹塞耳中，治积年耳聋。狂癫不能语、不识人者，和酒服三升良。

（四）皮：覆患疟人良。

（五）又，和毛煎，令作胶，治一切风毒骨节痛，呻吟不止者，消和酒服良。

（六）又，骨煮作汤，浴渍身，治历节风。

（七）又，煮头汁，令服三二升，治多年消渴，无不瘥者。

（八）又，脂和乌梅为丸，治多年疟。未发时服三十丸。

（九）又，头中一切风，以毛一斤炒令黄，投一斗酒中，渍三日。空心细细饮，使醉。衣覆卧取汗。明日更依前服。忌陈仓米、麦面等。

（十）卒心痛，绞结连腰脐者，取驴乳三升，热服之瘥。

## 110. Lü〔驴, donkey, Equus Asinus〕

Its meat is mainly used to treat madness and depression and quiet heart qi.

Dehair its head with boiling, boil it to make juice and soak the distiller's yeast in the juice to make liquor, which can be used to treat leprosy.

Mash up its raw fat with Shengjiao〔生椒, zanthoxylum, Zanthoxyli Pericarpium〕, wrap the paste with Mian〔绵, silk floss, Bombycis Lana〕and stuff it in ear to treat deafness for years. To treat a patient who is so mad that he can't speak or know the acquaintance, mix the paste with 3 Sheng of liquor and take it. It is quite effective.

It is quite effective in treating malaria by covering the patient with its hide.

Decoct its haired hide into glue to treat all kinds of pain in the joints caused by the wind evil which makes the patient moan all the time. Dissolve the glue and take it with liquor. It is quite effective.

Bathing in the boiled water with its bones can treat the joint-running wind.

Drinking 2 or 3 Sheng of the soup made by its boiled head can be used to treat consumptive thirst for years. The disease is certain to be cured.

Make its fat with Wumei〔乌梅, mume, Mume Fructus〕into pills to treat the malaria for years. Take thirty pills before the malaria occurs.

To treat all kinds of wind evils in the head, stir-fry 1 Jin of its hair until it turns yellow and put it into 1 Dou of liquor to soak for three days. Slowly drink the liquor on an empty stomach to be drunk and lie in bed with clothes on and quilt covered in order to sweat. The next day, drink the liquor according to the previous method. When drinking the liquor, don't eat Chencangmi〔陈仓米, old rice, Oryzae Semen Vetum〕and Maimian〔麦面, barley flour, Hordei Farina〕.

To treat the sudden pain in the heart which affects the waist and umbilicus, have a hot drink of 3 Sheng of Lüru〔驴乳, donkey's milk, Asini Lac〕. The disease will be cured.

# 111. 鸡

（一）（丹雄鸡）：主患白虎[1]，可铺饭于患处，使鸡食之良。又取热粪封之取热，使伏于患人床下。

（二）其肝入补肾方中，用冠血和天雄四分，桂心二分，太阳粉四分，丸服之，益阳气。

（三）乌雄鸡：主心痛，除心腹恶气。

（四）又，虚弱人取一只，治如食法。五味汁和肉一器中，封口，重汤中煮之，使骨肉相去即食之，甚补益。仍须空腹饱食之。肉须烂，生即反损。亦可五味腌，经宿，炙食之，分为两顿。

（五）又，刺在肉中不出者，取尾二七枚，烧作灰，以男子乳汁和封疮，刺当出。

（六）又，目泪出不止者，以三年冠血敷目睛上，日三度。

（七）乌雌鸡：温，味酸，无毒。主除风寒湿痹[2]，治反胃[3]、安胎及腹痛，踒折骨疼，乳痈[4]。

（八）月蚀疮[5]绕耳根，以乌雌鸡胆汁敷之，日三。

（九）产后血不止，以鸡子三枚，醋半升，好酒二升，煎取一升，分为四服。

如人行三二里[6],微暖进之。

（十）又,新产妇可取一只,理如食法,和五味炒熟,香,即投二升酒中,封口经宿,取饮之,令人肥白。

（十一）又,和乌油麻二升,熬令黄香,末之入酒,酒尽极效。(以乌油麻一升,熬之令香,末,和酒服之,即饱热能食。)

（十二）黄雌鸡:主腹中水癖[7]水肿,以一只理如食法:和赤小豆一升同煮,候豆烂即出食之。其汁,日二夜一,每服四合。补丈夫阳气,治冷气。瘦著床者,渐渐食之良。

（十三）又,先患骨热者,不可食之。鸡子动风气,不可多食。

（十四）又,光粉诸石为末,和饭与鸡食之,后取鸡食之,甚补益。

（十五）又,子醋煮熟,空腹食之,治久赤白痢。

（十六）又,人热毒发,可取三颗鸡子白,和蜜一合,服之瘥。

（十七）治大人及小儿发热,可取卵三颗,白蜜一合,相和服之,立瘥。卵并不得和蒜食,令人短气[8]。

（十八）又,胞衣不出,生吞鸡子清一枚,治目赤痛,除心胸伏热,烦满咳逆,动心气,不宜多食。

（十九）鸡具五色者,食之致狂。肉和鱼肉汁食之,成心瘕[9]。六指,玄鸡白头家鸡,及鸡死足爪不伸者,食并害人。

（二十）鸡子和葱,食之气短。鸡子白共鳖同食损人。鸡子共獭肉同食,成遁尸注[10],药不能治。

（二十一）鸡、兔同食成泄痢。小儿五岁已下,未断乳者,勿与鸡肉食。

【注释】

[1] 白虎:白虎历节,病症名,四肢关节走痛(疼痛游走不定),痛不可忍,不得屈伸的疾患,简称"历节",又名"痛风"。

[2] 风寒湿痹:病症名。风、寒、湿三气外邪侵袭经络,气血闭阻不畅引起。症状有肢体关节走窜疼痛,舌苔黄腻、脉浮、肌肤麻木等。

[3] 反胃:病症名。反胃,又称"胃反",是指饮食入胃、停滞不化、良久反出的病症。

[4] 乳痈:以乳房红肿疼痛,乳汁排出不畅,以致结脓成痈的急性化脓性病症,多发于产后哺乳的产妇,尤其是初产妇更为多见,俗称"奶疮"。

[5] 月蚀疮:又名"旋耳疮",指发生于耳根部的湿疮类疾病,可见于现代医学的外耳湿疹、耳后间擦性湿疹。

［6］里:中国长度计量单位,1 里等于 500 米。

［7］水癖:病症名,因水气结聚两胁而成癖病。癖病又称"癖气",指痞块生于两胁,平时寻摸不见,痛时则可触及。

［8］短气:指因呼吸短促而不相接续的情况。

［9］心痕:心下(胃口)生有结块。心下,中医学指膈下胃脘的部位。症痕是中医特有的病症名称,指腹中结块的病。坚硬不移动,痛有定处为症;聚散无常,痛无定处为痕。

［10］遁尸注:也称"遁尸",病症名,是一种突然发作、以心腹胀满刺痛、喘急为主症的危重病症。

## 111. Ji［鸡, chicken, Gallus Gallus Domesticus Brisson］

Red Xiongji［雄鸡, cock, Gallus Masculinus］is mainly used to treat the white tiger joint running[1]. Put the food in the affected part to make it peck. It is very effective. Apply hot droppings to the affected part to make the heat absorbed and let red Xiongji［雄鸡, cock, Gallus Masculinus］lie under the patient's bed.

Its liver is used in the formula for tonifying the kidney. The pills made with cockscomb blood, 4 Fen of Tianxiong［天雄, tianxiong aconite, Aconiti Radix Lateralis Tianxiong］, 2 Fen of Guixin［桂心, shaved cinnamon bark, Cinnamomi Cortex Rasus］and 4 Fen of sulphur can replenish yang qi.

Black Xiongji［雄鸡, cock, Gallus Masculinus］is mainly used to treat the pain in the heart and to eliminate malign qi in the heart and abdomen.

The person in poor health can prepare a black Xiongji［雄鸡, cock, Gallus Masculinus］for cooking as usual, put it in a container, add sauce to it, seal the container and boil the container in water until its bones and meat are separated. Eating it can benefit him greatly. It is necessary that the person should eat it on an empty stomach till he is full. It must be thoroughly cooked, otherwise it will be harmful to health. It can also be marinated in the sauce and the ordinary cooking seasonings for one night, stir-fried and eaten in two meals.

To treat the disease caused by the thorn deep in the flesh, burn fourteen feathers from the tail of Xiongji［雄鸡, cock, Gallus Masculinus］to ash, mix the ash with milk of the woman who gives birth to a boy and apply them to the

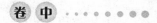

wound. The thorn will be pulled out easily.

To treat the tearing from eyes, apply the cockscomb blood of a three-year-old black Xiongji [雄鸡, cock, Gallus Masculinus] to the eyes three times every day.

The black hen, sour in taste and warm and non-toxic in property, is mainly used to eliminate the wind-cold dampness impediment[2], treat regurgitation[3] and breast carbuncle[4], prevent miscarriage, and relieve the abdominal pain and the pain in the sinews and bones caused by sprain and fracture.

To treat the ear-turning sore[5] behind ear, apply the bile of the black hen to the sore three times every day.

To treat the incessant postpartum bleeding, decoct three eggs of a black hen, half a Sheng of vinegar and 2 Sheng of good-quality liquor into 1 Sheng of decoction and take it in four times. The interval between each taking is about the time a person spends walking 2 or 3 Li[6]. Slightly heat it before taking it.

A woman who just delivers a baby can prepare a black hen for cooking as usual and stir-fry it with the ordinary cooking seasonings. When it is cooked and smells fragrant, put it into 2 Sheng of liquor, seal the container of the liquor for one night and drink the liquor next day, which can make her plump and white.

Decoct a black hen with 2 Sheng of Wuma [乌麻, black sesame, Sesami Semen Nigrum] until the hen turns yellow and smells fragrant, grind the hen and Wuma [乌麻, black sesame, Sesami Semen Nigrum] into powder and put the powder into the liquor. Completely drinking the liquor will be extremely effective. Decoct a black hen with 1 Sheng of Wuma [乌麻, black sesame, Sesami Semen Nigrum] to make the hen smell fragrant, grind the hen and Wuma [乌麻, black sesame, Sesami Semen Nigrum] into powder and take the powder with liquor, which can make one feel full and hot and eat more.

The yellow hen is mainly used to treat the water aggregation[7] and edema in abdomen. Prepare a yellow hen for cooking as usual, boil the hen with 1 Sheng of Chixiaodou [赤小豆, rice bean, Phaseoli Semen], take the hen out to eat when the beans are mashed and drink 4 Ge of the soup two times during the day and one time during the night, which can replenish the men's yang qi and treat cold qi. A bedridden, thin and weak patient can gradually eat the yellow hen, which is effective.

Those who suffered from heat in the bones shouldn't eat the yellow hen. The eggs of yellow hen will stir wind qi, so don't eat it excessively.

Grind Qianfen [铅粉, processed galenite, Galenitum Praeparatum] and all kinds of stone drugs into powder, feed the powder with rice to the yellow hen and eat the hen later, which is greatly beneficial.

Eating boiled eggs of yellow hen with vinegar on an empty stomach can treat the chronic red and white dysentery.

A patient who is attacked by the heat toxin can take three Jidanbai [鸡蛋白, egg white, Galli Albumen] of yellow hen with 1 Ge of honey. The disease will be cured.

To treat fever in adults and children, eat three eggs of yellow hen with 1 Ge of honey. The disease will be cured at once. Don't eat eggs with garlic, otherwise it will cause the shortness of breath[8].

A woman who just delivers a baby with the retention of the placenta can swallow an uncooked Jidanbai [鸡蛋白, egg white, Galli Albumen] of the yellow hen, which can also treat the redness and pain of the eyes and cough with dyspnea and upward counterflow of qi, and eliminate the latent heat in the chest and cease the vexation and fullness in the chest. But it can also stir heart qi, so don't eat it excessively.

Eating Ji [鸡, chicken, Gallus Gallus Domesticus Brisson] with colorful feathers can make people mad. Eating its meat with fish soup can lead to the epigastrium conglomeration[9]. Don't eat the one with six toes, the black one with a white head or the dead one without claws stretching out, for eating it is harmful to people.

Eating eggs with Cong [葱, scallion, Allii Fistulosi Herba] will cause the shortness of breath. Eating Jidanbai [鸡蛋白, egg white, Galli Albumen] with Bie [鳖, turtle, Trionyx Sinensis] will damage people's health. Eating eggs with the meat of Ta [獭, otter, Lutra Lutra] will cause Dunshi[10], which can't be cured by drugs.

Eating chicken with the meat of Tu [兔, rabbit, Oryctolagus Cuniculus] will cause diarrhea and dysentery. Don't let the unweaned children under five years old eat chicken.

# [ Notes ]

[ 1 ] white tiger joint running: A kind of disease which is the same as joint-running wind. The disease gets the name because it usually occurs from 3 a. m. to 5 a. m. This period is called "yin-period" (寅时) in China and "yin" (寅) means "tiger" in the twelve Chinese zodiac. The disease is characterized by the severe migratory pain in limbs and inability to bend and stretch. It is also called pain wind or gout in the Western medicine.

[ 2 ] wind-cold dampness impediment: A kind of disease caused by the invasion of wind, cold and dampness into the collaterals which results in the obstruction of qi and blood. The symptoms include the pain in the joints, the yellow and greasy tongue fur, the floating pulse, the numbness of the skin and so on.

[ 3 ] regurgitation: A kind of disease that the food in the stomach is not digested but is spit out after some time.

[ 4 ] breast carbuncle: A kind of disease characterized by the pain, the redness and swelling of the breast and the poor secretion of milk, which results in the acute suppurative disease of the breast caused by the pus becoming the carbuncle. It is more common among the puerperal breastfeeding women, especially primiparas. It is also known as mastitis.

[ 5 ] ear-turning sore: It is also known as the eczema of the ear or the intertrigo behind the ear. It is a kind of wet sore disease in the root of ear. In the modern medicine it is also called the eczema of external auditory meatus or the interstitial eczema behind the ear.

[ 6 ] Li: A unit of length in China. 1 Li is equal to 500 meters.

[ 7 ] water aggregation: An aggregation disease caused by water qi gathering in both sides of the chest. The aggregation disease refers to the fact that there are lumps in both sides of the chest and people can't feel the lumps in the normal times unless people are in pain.

[ 8 ] shortness of breath: The short, hasty, discontinuous breathing.

[ 9 ] epigastrium conglomeration: The lumps in the gastral cavity. Concretion and conglomeration are the unique disease names of TCM, referring to the disease of lumps in the abdomen. Concretion refers to the fact that the lump is hard and fixed, and the pain is also fixed, and conglomeration refers to the fact that the lump as well

as the pain is migratory.

[10] Dunshi: A critical disease characterized by the sudden attack, distention and fullness and severe pain in the heart and abdomen, and rapid panting.

# 112. 鹅

（一）脂：可合面脂。

（二）肉：性冷，不可多食。令人易霍乱。与服丹石人相宜。亦发痼疾。

（三）卵：温。补五藏，亦补中益气。多发痼疾。

# 112. E［鹅, goose, Anser Domestica Geese］

Its fat can be compounded into face cream.

Its meat is cold in property, so don't eat it excessively or it is likely to cause cholera. The person who takes Danshi is suitable to eat the meat. It can also cause the old intractable disease.

Its egg, warm in property, can be used to tonify the five zang-organs and the middle and replenish qi. It can often cause the old intractable disease.

# 113. 蜜 微温

（一）主心腹邪气，诸惊痫，补五藏不足气。益中止痛，解毒。能除众病，和百药，养脾气，除心烦闷，不能饮食。

（二）治心肚痛，血刺腹痛及赤白痢，则生捣地黄汁，和蜜一大匙，服即下。

（三）又，长服之，面如花色，仙方中甚贵此物。若觉热，四肢不和，即服蜜浆一碗，甚良。

（四）又能止肠澼，除口疮，明耳目，久服不饥。

（五）又，点目中热膜，家养白蜜为上，木蜜次之，崖蜜更次。

（六）又，治癫，可取白蜜一斤，生姜三斤捣取汁。先秤铜铛[1]，令知斤两。即下蜜于铛中消之。又秤，知斤两，下姜汁于蜜中，微火煎，令姜汁尽。秤蜜，斤两在即休，药已成矣。患三十年癫者，平旦服枣许大一丸，一日三服，酒饮任下。忌生冷醋滑臭物。功用甚多，世人众委，不能一一具之。

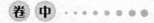

【注释】

[1] 铛:温器,似锅,三足。

## 113. Mi［蜜, honey, Mel］ *slightly warm*

It is mainly used to treat the evil qi in the heart and abdomen and all kinds of fright epilepsies, and supplement the insufficient qi of the five zang-organs. It is also used to tonify the middle, relieve pain, resolve toxin, treat all kinds of diseases, harmonize one hundred drugs, nourish spleen qi, eliminate the vexation and oppression in the heart and chest which robs the patient of the desire to drink and eat.

To treat the pain in the heart and abdomen, the abdominal pain caused by stagnation of blood, and red and white dysentery, crush Xiandihuang［鲜地黄, fresh rehmannia, Rehmanniae Radicis Recens］to extract the juice and drink it with a big spoon of honey, the disease will be cured.

Long-term taking of it will make the face look as beautiful as a flower. It is highly valued in the formulas of cultivating immortality. If feeling fever and being unwell in the limbs, drink one bowl of honey water at once. It is very effective.

It is used to treat dysentery and mouth sore, and improve hearing and vision. Long-term taking of it will make people feel no hunger.

To remove the pterygium, the honey made by domestic bees is the best, the wild one gotten from the beehives in the trees is next only to it, followed by the wild one gotten from the beehives in the mountains and cliffs.

To treat leprosy, crush 1 Jin of honey and 3 Jin of Shengjiang［生姜, fresh ginger, Zingiberis Rhizoma Recens］to extract the juice. First weigh the copper Cheng[1] to know its weight and put the honey into the Cheng to dissolve it. Then weigh the Cheng again to know the weight and put the juice into the Cheng to mix with the honey, and decoct them with small fire until the juice runs out. Weigh the honey, and if it weighs the same as before, the medicine is made. The patient suffering from leprosy for thirty years can take a pill with the size of a Dazao［大枣, jujube, Jujubae Fructus］at ordinary times and take it three times a day with liquor or rice soup. The patient is forbidden to eat the raw, cold, sour, slippery, rotten and stinky food. People know that it has many effects which can't be listed in detail.

【Note】

[1] Cheng: A three-legged and pan-like heater which can be used for decocting herbs.

# 114. 牡 蛎

（一）火上炙，令沸。去壳食之，甚美。令人细润肌肤，美颜色。

（二）又，药家比来取左顾者，若食之，即不拣左右也。可长服之。海族之中，惟此物最贵。北人不识，不能表其味尔。

## 114. Muli〔牡蛎，oyster，Ostrea Gigas Thunberg〕

Stir-fry it to make its juice boil and overflow from its shell. Remove its shell to eat, and it tastes very delicious. It can make people's skin smooth and soft and make people look beautiful.

In the past, the people who dealt with medicinal materials chose left Mulike〔牡蛎壳，oyster shell，Ostreae Concha〕as a kind of medicinal material. To eat Muli〔牡蛎，oyster，Ostrea Gigas Thunberg〕it doesn't matter whether the shell is left or right. It can be eaten frequently. It is the most valuable in the seafood. Northerners don't know it so they cannot tell its taste.

# 115. 龟 甲 温

（一）味酸。主除温瘴气，风痹，身肿，踒折。又，骨带入山林中，令人不迷路。其食之法，一如鳖法也。其中黑色者，常啖蛇，不中食之。其壳亦不堪用。

（二）其甲：能主女人漏下赤白、崩中，小儿囟不合，破症瘕、痎疟，疗五痔，阴蚀，湿痹[1]，女子阴隐疮及骨节中寒热，煮汁浴渍之良。

（三）又，已前都用水中龟，不用啖蛇龟。五月五日取头干末服之，亦令人长远入山不迷。

（四）又方，卜师处钻了者，涂酥炙，细罗，酒下二钱，疗风疾[2]。

【注释】

[1] 湿痹：病症名，痹病中的一种，又名"肌痹"，因风寒湿三邪中以湿邪偏

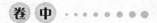

胜、湿性黏腻滞着所致,表现为肌肤麻木、关节重着、肿痛处固定不移。

[2] 风疾:指风痹、半身不遂等症。

### 115. Guijia [龟甲, tortoise shell and plastron, Testudinis Carapax et Plastrum] *warm*

Sour in taste, it is mainly used to eliminate the warm evil, resolve miasma, and treat the wind impediment, generalized swelling and sprain and the fracture of the sinews and bones. People will not get lost in the mountains and forests while bringing the bones of Gui [龟, tortoise, Tesudines]. The way of eating Gui [龟, tortoise, Tesudines] is the same as the way of eating Bie [鳖, turtle, Trionyx Sinensis]. Black Gui [龟, tortoise, Tesudines] often eats snakes which makes it inedible. Its shell and plastron can't be used for medicinal materials.

Guijia [龟甲, tortoise shell and plastron, Testudinis Carapax et Plastrum] is mainly used to treat red and white vaginal discharge in women, profuse vaginal bleeding, infantile metopism, abdominal mass, malaria, five kinds of hemorrhoids, vulva ulcer and dampness impediment[1]. Bathing in the boiled water with its shell and plastron, it is effective in treating the women who suffer from vulva ulcer and hemorrhoids and cold and heat in the joints of bones.

In the past Gui [龟, tortoise, Tesudines] living in the water instead of the one eating snakes was used as medicinal materials. On the fifth day of the fifth lunar month, dry its head, grind it into powder and take it, making people not get lost in the deep mountains and forests as well.

To treat the wind disease[2], take the burnt Guijia [龟甲, tortoise shell and plastron, Testudinis Carapax et Plastrum] from the diviner, spread it with Su [酥, butter, Bovis seu Ovis Butyrum], broil it, pound it into powder, sieve it to make finer and take 2 Qian of the powder.

【Notes】

[1] dampness impediment: One kind of impediment diseases, also known as the impediment of flesh, caused by the invasion of wind, cold and dampness, especially by the sticky, slimy and inhibited dampness. It is characterized by the numbness of skin, heavy and difficult to stretch joints, and the fixed swelling and pain.

[2] wind disease: The disease such as wind impediment, hemiplegia and so on.

# 116. 魁 蛤 寒

润五藏,治消渴,开关节。服丹石人
食之,使人免有疮肿及热毒所生也。

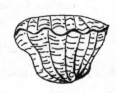

## 116. Kuige [魁蛤, sea clam, Cyclina Sinensis] *cold*

It is used to nourish the five zang-organs, treat the consumptive thirst and make the joints flexible. People taking Danshi and eating it won't suffer from the swollen sore and other diseases caused by the heat toxin.

# 117. 鳢鱼(蠡鱼)

（一）下大小便壅塞气。

（二）又,作脍,与脚气风气人食
之,效。

（三）又,以大者洗去泥,开肚,
以胡椒末半两,切大蒜三两颗,内鱼
腹中缝合,并和小豆一升煮之。临熟

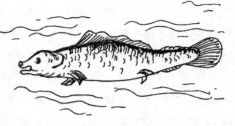

下萝蔔三五颗如指大,切葱一握,煮熟。空腹食之,并豆等强饱,尽食之。至夜
即泄气无限,三五日更一顿。下一切恶气。

（四）又,十二月作酱,良也。

## 117. Liyu (Liyu) [鳢鱼(蠡鱼), snakehead mullet, Ophiocephalus Argus Cantor]

It is used to descend the congested qi which causes the difficulty in urination and defecation.

Cutting it into thin slices, and eating the slices is effective to treat people suffering from weak foot and wind qi.

Take a big one, wash the mud from it, cut its belly open, put half a Liang of the powder of Hujiao〔胡椒, pepper, Piperis Fructus〕and two or three pieces of the chopped garlic into the belly, sew it up and cook it with 1 Sheng of Chixiaodou〔赤小豆, rice bean, Phaseoli Semen〕. When it's about to be thoroughly cooked, put three or five finger-sized Luobo〔萝卜, radish, Raphani Radix〕and a handful of chopped Cong〔葱, scallion, Allii Fistulosi Herba〕into the pot. After it is cooked, eat it with Chixiaodou〔赤小豆, rice bean, Phaseoli Semen〕up on an empty stomach until it is quite full. At night there will be incessant aerofluxus. Eat another meal in three or five days, and all malign qi will be eliminated.

The fish paste made of it in the twelfth lunar month is of good quality.

## 118. 鲇鱼（鳑鱼）、鳠（鮠鱼）

鲇与鳠大约相似,主诸补益,无鳞,有毒,勿多食。赤目、赤须者并杀人也。

## 118. Nianyu（Yiyu）, Hu（Weiyu）〔鲇鱼（鳑鱼）、鳠（鮠鱼）, catfish, channel catfish, Parasilurus Asotus, Leiocassis Longirostris Günther〕

Nianyu〔鲇鱼, catfish, Parasilurus Asotus〕, similar to Hu〔鳠, channel catfish, Leiocassis Longirostris Günther〕, is mainly used for tonifying. Without scales, it is toxic in property, so don't eat it excessively. Eating the one with red eyes and red whiskers can poison people to death.

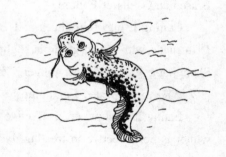

## 119. 鲫 鱼

（一）食之平胃气,调中,益五藏,和莼作羹食良。

（二）作脍食之,断暴下痢。和蒜食之,有少热;和姜酱食之,有少冷。

（三）又，夏月热痢可食之，多益。冬月则不治也。

（四）骨：烧为灰，敷恶疮上，三、五次瘥。

（五）又，鲫鱼与鳜[1]，其状颇同，味则有殊。鳜是节化[2]。鲫是稷米化之[4]，其鱼肚上尚有米色。宽大者是鲫，背高肚狭小者是鳜，其功不及鲫鱼。

（六）谨按：其子调中，益肝气[3]。凡鱼生子，皆粘在草上及土中。寒冬月水过后，亦不腐坏。每到五月三伏时，雨中便化为鱼。

（七）食鲫鱼不得食沙糖，令人成疳虫。丹石热毒发者，取荽首和鲫鱼作羹，食一两顿即瘥。

**【注释】**

[1] 鳜：一种鱼，似鲫而小，薄而黑。

[2] 鳜是节化："节"有说为"栉"。节为竹节；栉为梳子、篦子等梳头发的用具。古人认为，"鳜是节化"（鳜鱼是节变化而成）以及下文所说"鲫是稷米化之"都是一种错误认识。

[3] 肝气：指肝脏之精气与功能。

### 119. Jiyu［鲫鱼, crucian, Carassius Auratus］

Eating it can calm stomach qi, regulate the middle and tonify the five zang-organs. It's effective to make fish soup with Chuncai［莼菜, water shield, Braseniae Caulis et Folium］.

Cutting it into thin slices and eating the slices can cure the acute dysentery. Dish made with it and garlic is slightly hot in property while dish made with it and Shengjiang［生姜, fresh ginger, Zingiberis Rhizoma Recens］and Doubanjiang［豆瓣酱, bean paste, Leguminosae Pasta］is slightly cold in property.

Eating it in summer is effective in treating the heat dysentery while eating it in winter is not effective in treating dysentery.

Burn the bones to ash and apply it to the severe sore, and the sore will be cured after three or five times.

It is quite similar to Jie fish[1] in appearance but different in taste. The Jie fish develops from bamboo joints while it develops from Jimi[2]［稷米, non-glutinous broomcorn millet, Panici Non-Glutinosi Semen］with millet-like color in the belly. It has a large body while Jie fish has a high back and small belly. The effect of Jie fish is not as good as that of it.

The following is supplemented by Zhang Ding: Its roes can be used to regulate the middle and replenish liver qi[3]. When it spawns, its roes will stick to grass and soil. In winter, its roes won't rot, and even they are soaked in cold water. During dog days in the fifth lunar month its roes will become fish in the rain.

Don't eat it with Shatang [沙糖, granulated sugar, Saccharon Granulatum], or people will have Gan worms in the body. A person attacked by the heat toxin of Danshi can make fish soup with it and Jiaoshou [菱首, infested ear of wild rice, Zizaniae Spica Infestata], and the toxin will be resolved after one or two times of taking.

**【Notes】**

[1] Jie fish: A kind of fish which is similar to the crucian but smaller. Compared to crucian it is black and thinner.

[2] The Jie fish develops from bamboo joints while it develops from Jimi: The ancient people had a wrong idea that the Jie fish developed from the bamboo joints while the crucian developed from the non-glutinous broomcorn millets.

[3] liver qi: The essence and function of the liver.

# 120. 鳝鱼(黄鳝)

补五藏,逐十二风邪。患恶气人当作臛,空腹饱食,便以衣盖卧。少顷当汗出如白胶,汗从腰脚中出。候汗尽,暖五木[1]汤浴,须慎风一日。更三、五日一服,并治湿风。

**【注释】**

[1] 五木:柳树枝、桃树枝、榆树枝、桑树枝和女贞树枝。

## 120. Shanyu (Huangshan) [鳝鱼(黄鳝), eel, Monopterus Albus]

It is used to tonify the five zang-organs and expel twelve kinds of wind evils. Those suffering the malign qi can make fish soup with it, eat their fill on an empty stomach and lie in bed with clothes on and quilts covered in order to sweat. After a while sweat will come out of the waist and legs like white glues. After sweating, they should bathe in the hot five-wood[1] water. After bathing, they must avoid exposure to wind for a day. Do it again in three or five days. It can also be used to treat rheumatism.

【Note】

[1] five-wood: The five kinds of tree branches are willow branches, peach branches, elm branches, mulberry branches and privet branches.

# 121. 鲤 鱼

（一）胆：主除目中赤及热毒痛，点之良。

（二）肉：白煮食之，疗水肿脚满，下气。腹中有宿瘕不可食，害人。久服天门冬人，亦不可食。

（三）刺在肉中，中风水肿痛者，烧鲤鱼眼睛作灰，内疮中，汁出即可。

（四）谨按：鱼血主小儿丹毒[1]，涂之即瘥。

（五）鱼鳞：烧，烟绝，研。酒下方寸（匕），破产妇滞血。

（六）脂：主诸痫，食之良。

（七）肠：主小儿腹中疮。

（八）鲤鱼鲊[2]：不得和豆藿叶食之，成瘦。

（九）其鱼子，不得合猪肝食之。

（十）又，（凡修理），每断去脊上两筋及脊内黑血，此是毒故也。

（十一）炙鲤鱼切忌烟，不得令熏着眼，损人眼光。三两日内必见验也。

（十二）又，天行病后不可食，再发即死。

（十三）又，（其在）砂石中者，（有）毒，多在脑髓中，不可食其头。

【注释】

[1] 丹毒：病症名，是指以皮肤突然发红成片、色如涂丹为主要表现的急性感染性疾病。

[2] 鲊：一种用盐和红曲腌的鱼。

## 121. Liyu［鲤鱼, carp, Cyprinus Carpio］

Its bile is mainly used to treat the redness of eyes and the pain of eyes caused by the heat toxin. It is effective in putting drops of its bile in eyes.

Boil its meat with water to eat it to treat the edema and foot swelling, and promote qi to descend. Those who suffer from the old intractable conglomeration disease shouldn't eat it as it will be harmful to health. Those who have a long-term taking of Tianmendong〔天门冬, asparagus, Asparagi Radix〕shouldn't eat it either.

To treat the swelling and pain resulting from the infection of wind and water caused by the thorns deep in the flesh, burn its eyes to ash and put the ash in the wound. It will be cured after pus is expelled.

The following is supplemented by Zhang Ding: Its blood is mainly used to treat the erysipelas[1] in children. It will be cured after applying its blood to it.

Burn its scales until smoke is gone and grind them into powder. Taking 1 Fangcunbi (square-cun-spoon) of the powder with liquor can eliminate the blood stasis in a woman who just delivers a baby.

Its fat is mainly used to treat all kinds of epilepsies. Eating it is effective.

Its intestines are mainly used to treat the sores in children's abdomen.

Don't eat fish Zha[2] of it with the leaves of Dadou〔大豆, soybean, Sojae Semen〕because it can make people lose weight.

Don't eat its roes with Zhugan〔猪肝, pig's liver, Suis Iecur〕.

While preparing it for cooking, remove the two sinews and black blood in its back because they are toxic.

While broiling it, avoid smoke going into eyes because it will damage the vision. If smoke goes into eyes, the vision will be damaged in two or three days.

Recovering from the epidemic, don't eat it or it will cause people to die when the epidemic recurs.

The one living under sand and gravel of water is toxic, and mostly its toxin is in brain, so don't eat its head.

【Notes】

[1] erysipelas: An acute infectious disease characterized by the sudden redness in patches of skin and the red is like the color smeared with cinnabar.

[2] Zha: The fish salted with the red infested rice.

# 122. 鳖

（一）主妇人漏下，羸瘦。仲春食之美，夏月有少腥气。

（二）其甲：岳州[1]昌江[2]者为上。赤足不可食，杀人。

【注释】

[1]岳州：古地名，今湖南省洞庭湖周围东、南、北一带地方。

[2]昌江：古地名，在今江西省东北部一带。

## 122. Bie〔鳖, turtle, Trionyx Sinensis〕

It is mainly used to treat the vaginal bleeding in women, weakness and emaciation. It tastes delicious in the second month of spring and fishy in summer.

It is the most effective to use Biejia〔鳖甲, turtle shell, Trionycis Carapax〕 produced in Yuezhou[1] and Changjiang[2]. Bie〔鳖, turtle, Trionyx Sinensis〕 with the red feet is inedible which can poison people to death.

〔Notes〕

[1] Yuezhou：A name of a place in ancient China. It is mainly the area around the east, south and north of Dongting Lake in Hunan Province now.

[2] Changjiang：A name of a place in ancient China. It is the area in the northeast of Jiangxi Province now.

# 123. 蟹

（一）足斑、目赤不可食，杀人。

（二）主散诸热。（又堪）治胃气，理经脉，消食。

（三）蟹脚中髓及脑，能续断筋骨。人取蟹脑髓，微熬之，令内疮中，筋即连续。

（四）又，八月前，每个蟹腹内有稻谷一颗，用输海神。待输芒[1]后，过八月方食即好。（未输时为长未成）。经霜更美，未经霜时有毒。

（五）又，盐淹之作蝑，有气味。和酢食之，利肢节，去五藏中烦闷气。其物虽恶形容，食之甚益人。

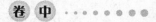

（六）爪：能安胎。

【注释】

［1］输芒：传说蟹于八月稻熟时腹中有一稻芒，献于海神。输就是"输送，捐献"。

### 123. Xie ［蟹, crab, Brachyura］

The one with spots on its legs or red eyes is inedible because it can poison people to death.

It is mainly used to dissipate all kinds of heat. It is also used to treat the stomach qi, regulate the meridians and promote the digestion.

Its marrow in legs and brain can be used to remedy the severe injury of the sinews and bones. Decoct slightly its marrow or brain, put it into wound, and then the injury of the sinews and bones will be remedied.

Before the eighth lunar month, there is a grain of rice in its belly which will be dedicated to the God of the sea (commonly known as "Shumang"[1]). People should wait to eat it after the eighth lunar month when it experiences Shumang. (The crab that has not experienced Shumang is not grown up.) It will become more delicious after frost, and it is toxic in property if it is not after frost.

The salted paste smells terrible, and it should be eaten with the vinegar which can make the joints flexible and eliminate the vexation and oppression in the five zang-organs. It looks ugly and fierce, but in fact eating it can benefit people greatly.

Its claw can be used to prevent miscarriage.

【Note】

［1］Shumang: In ancient China, a legend said that there was a grain of rice in the crab's belly in the eighth lunar month when rice riped. The grain would be dedicated to the God of the sea. The dedication of the grain to the God of the sea was called "Shumang".

### 124. 乌贼鱼

（一）食之少有益髓。

（二）骨：主小儿、大人下痢，炙令黄，去皮细研成粉，粥中调服之良。

（三）其骨能消目中一切浮瞖[1]。细研和蜜点之妙。

（四）又,骨末治眼中热泪[2]。又,点马眼热泪甚良。

（五）久食之,主绝嗣无子,益精。其鱼腹中有墨一片,堪用书字。

**【注释】**

［1］浮瞖:"瞖"同"翳"。翳为眼球上生的障蔽视线的翳膜。浮瞖为表浅的翳膜,容易剥离。

［2］热泪:病症名,指目中多泪,泪下热感,或泪热如汤,伴目睛红赤、肿痛、羞明等症。

### 124. Wuzeiyu［乌贼鱼, Cuttlefish, Sepia Esculenta Hoyle］

Eating it can slightly replenish the essence and marrow.

Its bones are mainly used to treat the dysentery in children and adults. Broil its bones until they turn yellow, remove its epidermis, grind it into fine powder and put it in the gruel to eat. It is effective.

Its bones can be used to eliminate all kinds of floating nebulas[1] in eyes. Grind it into fine powder and put it in eyes with honey. It is quite effective.

The powder made by its bones is used to treat the heat tearing[2]. It is quite effective in treating the heat tearing of a horse by putting powder in its eyes.

Long-term taking of it is mainly used to treat infertility and replenish essence. There is ink in its stomach which can be used for writing.

**【Notes】**

［1］floating nebulas: Nebula is a screen that covers the eyeball and can obstruct the view. The floating nebula is the superficial screen in the eye and can be easy to remove.

［2］heat tearing: A kind of eye disease. It has the symptoms of tearing, hot tears which are as hot as hot soup, red eyes, swelling and pain in the eyes, being afraid of light, etc.

### 125. 白　鱼

（一）主肝家不足气,不堪多食,泥人心。虽不发病,终养虿所食[1]。

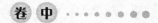

（二）和豉作羹,一两顿而已。新鲜者好食。若经宿者不堪食。（久食）令人腹冷生诸疾。或淹、或糟藏,犹可食。

（三）又可炙了,于葱、醋中重煮（一两沸）食之。调五藏,助脾气,能消食。理十二经络,舒展不相及气。

（四）时人好作饼,炙食之。犹少动气,久亦不损人也。

【注释】

[1] 养蚛所食:养的意思是"提供"。蚛就是蚛虫,一种肉眼看不见的很小的寄生虫。养蚛所食意思是"提供蚛虫所需要的食物"。

### 125. Baiyu [白鱼, topmouth culter, Erythroculter Ilishaeformis]

It is mainly used to supplement insufficient qi of the liver. Don't eat it excessively, or it will weaken heart qi. Although it will not cause diseases, it will eventually provide food for the ni worms[1].

It is enough to have one or two meals of fish soup made of it and Douchi [豆豉, fermented soybean, Sojae Semen Fermentatum]. The fresh one is tasty while the overnight one is inedible. Long-term eating of it will make people feel cold in abdomen and suffer from many diseases. It is edible if stored after being salted or marinated in liquor or Jiuzao [酒糟, liquor dregs, Vini Residuum].

Stir-frying it, boiling it with Cong [葱, scallion, Allii Fistulosi Herba] and vinegar for one or two times and eating it can regulate the five zang-organs, improve spleen qi, promote digestion, regulate the twelve channels and free qi that are not meant to be connected.

Nowadays, people like to make cakes with it and bake them to eat. This way of eating can slightly stir qi, but long-term eating won't damage people's health.

【Note】

[1] ni worms: Tiny parasites that are invisible to the naked eyes.

### 126. 鳜 鱼 平

补劳,益脾胃。稍有毒。

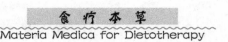
**126. Guiyu〔鳜鱼, mandarin fish, Siniperca Chuatsi〕** *mild*

It is used to supplement deficiency due to overstrain and fortify the spleen and stomach. It is slightly toxic in property.

## 127. 青　鱼

（一）主脚气烦闷。又,和韭白煮食之,治脚气脚弱、烦闷、益心力也。

（二）又,头中有枕,取之蒸,令气通,曝干,状如琥珀。此物疗卒心痛,平水气。以水研服之良。

（三）又,胆、眼睛:益人眼,取汁注目中,主目暗。亦涂热疮,良。

**127. Qingyu〔青鱼, black carp, Mylopharyngodon Piceus〕**

It is mainly used to treat the vexation and oppression in the heart and chest caused by weak foot. Boil it with the stalk of Jiucai〔韭菜, Chinese leek, Allii Tuberosi Folium〕and eat it to treat the weak feet and the vexation and oppression in the heart and chest caused by weak foot, and to keep people mentally and physically fit.

There is an occipital bone in its head. Take the bone, steam it until the steam goes upward and dry it in the sun. It looks like Hupo〔琥珀, amber, Succinum〕. It can be used to treat the sudden pain in the heart and expel the water qi. It is effective to take it after it is ground with water.

Its bile and eyes can benefit people's eyes. Put drops of bile or eye juice in people's eyes to treat the dim vision. It is also effective in treating the heat sore by the external application.

## 128. 石首鱼（黄花鱼）

作干鲞,消宿食,主中恶,不堪鲜食。

## 128. Shishouyu（Huanghuayu）[石首鱼（黄花鱼），drumfish（yellow croaker），Pseudosciaena Crocea aut Psendosciaena Polyactis]

Its dried salty fillet can be used to remove the retention of undigested food and treat the malignity stroke. The fresh one can't be eaten raw.

## 129. 嘉 鱼 微温

常于崖石下孔中吃乳石沫，甚补益。微有毒。其味甚珍美也。

## 129. Jiayu [嘉鱼，Prenant's schizothoracin，Schizothorax Prenanti] *slightly warm*

It often eats the foams of Zhongrushi [钟乳石，stalactite，Stalactitumin] in the stone caves under cliff. It can benefit people greatly. It is slightly toxic in property and very delicious.

## 130. 鲈 鱼[1] 平

（一）主安胎，补中。作脍尤佳。

（二）补五藏，益筋骨，和肠胃，治水气。多食宜人。作鲊犹良。

（三）又，暴干甚香美。虽有小毒，不至发病。

【注释】

[1]鲈鱼：中文里有许多种鱼类都可以被称为"鲈鱼"，其中最常见的有四种，分别是：海鲈鱼，学名"日本真鲈"，分布于近海及河口海水淡水交汇处；松江鲈鱼，也称"四鳃鲈鱼"，属于降海洄游鱼类，最为著名；大口黑鲈，也称"加州鲈鱼"，从美国引进的新品种；河鲈，也称"赤鲈""五道黑"，原产新疆北部地区。文章中所指鲈鱼应为第一种。

## 130. Luyu[1] [鲈鱼, common sea perch, Lateolabrax Japonicus] *mild*

It is mainly used to prevent miscarriage and tonify the middle. The cut slices are especially effective.

It is used to tonify the five zang-organs, strengthen the sinews and bones, harmonize the stomach and intestines and treat the water qi disease. Regular eating of it can benefit people. It is especially effective to make fish Zha of it.

Its dried fillet is very delicious. Though it is slightly toxic in property, it doesn't cause diseases.

【Note】

[1] There are many kinds of fish in Chinese that can be called perch, among which the following four kinds are the most common. The first one is Hailuyu [海鲈鱼, common sea perch, Lateolabrax Japonicus], which lives near the coastal waters and river mouth waters of the intersection of fresh water and sea water. The second kind is Songjiang Luyu [松江鲈鱼, roughskin sculpin, Trachidermus Fasciatus], also known as four-gill bass, which is the most famous and is a kind of catadromous migration fish. The third kind is Dakou Heilu [大口黑鲈, largemouth black bass, Micropterus Salmoides], also known as California sea bass, is a new species introduced from the United States. The fourth kind is Helu [河鲈, river bass, Perca Fluviatilis Linnaeus], also known as Chilu (赤鲈) and Wudaohei (五道黑), which is native to northern Xinjiang. The perch mentioned in this article should be the first kind.

## 131. 比目鱼 平

补虚,益气力。多食稍动气。

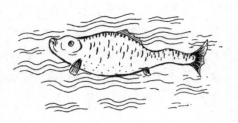

## 131. Bimuyu [比目鱼, flatfish, Pleuronectiformes aut Heterosomata] *mild*

It can be used to supplement deficiency and replenish qi and energy. Eating it excessively can slightly stir qi.

## 132. 鯸鮧鱼（河豚）

（一）有毒，不可食之。其肝毒杀人。缘腹中无胆，头中无鳃，故知害人。若中此毒及鲈鱼毒者，便锉芦根煮汁饮，解之。

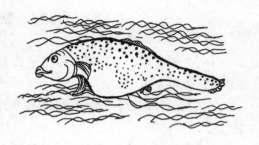

（二）又，此鱼行水之次，或自触着物，即自怒气胀，浮于水上，为鸦鹞所食。

### 132. Houyiyu (Hetun)〔鯸鮧鱼（河豚），puffer，Tetraodontidae〕

It is toxic in property, so it is inedible. The toxin in the liver can poison people to death. Because there is no gall in the stomach and no gills in the head, it can be deduced that it is harmful to people. The poisoning from eating it or Luyu〔鲈鱼，common sea perch，Lateolabrax Japonicus〕can be resolved by drinking the boiled juice of chopped Lugen〔芦根，phragmites，Phragmitis Rhizoma〕.

When it swims in water, it may touch something. Then it will become angry, and its body will become round. And it will float over the water which makes it be eaten by some birds such as Wuya〔乌鸦，crow，Corvi Macrorhynchi Caro〕，Yao〔鹞，sparrow hawk，Accipiter Nisus〕and so on.

## 133. 黄鱼（鳣鱼）平

有毒。发诸气病，不可多食。亦发疮疥，动风。不宜和荞麦同食，令人失音也。

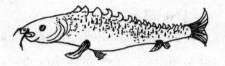

### 133. Huangyu (Zhanyu)〔黄鱼（鳣鱼），northern snakehead，Huso Dauricus〕mild

It is toxic in property. Don't eat it excessively or it will cause all kinds of qi diseases. It can also cause sores and scabies and stir wind. Don't eat it with Qiaomai［荞麦, buckwheat, Fagopyri Semen］, or it will cause the loss of voice.

## 134. 鲂 鱼

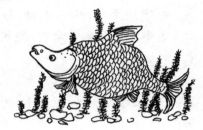

（一）调胃气,利五藏。和芥子酱食之,助肺气,去胃家风[1]。

（二）消谷不化者,作脍食,助脾气,令人能食。

（三）患疳痢者,不得食。作羹臛食,宜人。其功与鲫鱼同。

【注释】

［1］胃家风:胃家就是胃;胃家风就是胃风,即风邪中于胃者,以腹胀、泄下、多汗、恶风为特征。

## 134. Fangyu［鲂鱼, black bream, Megalobrama Skolkovii］

It is used to harmonize stomach qi and regulate the five zang-organs. Eating it with Jiecai［芥菜, mustard leaf, Sinapis Folium］sauce can improve lung qi and eliminate the stomach wind[1].

To treat indigestion, slice it and eat it, which can improve spleen qi and increase the appetite.

Patients suffering from the Gan dysentery shouldn't eat it. Its thick soup can benefit people. It has the same effect as Jiyu［鲫鱼, crucian, Carassius Auratus］.

【Note】

［1］stomach wind: A disease caused by wind evil invading the stomach. It is characterized by abdominal distention, diarrhea, sweating and aversion to wind.

## 135. 牡鼠（鼠）

（一）主小儿痫疾[1]、腹大贪食者:可以黄泥裹烧之。细拣去骨,取肉和五味汁作羹与食之。勿令食着骨,甚瘦人。

（二）又，取腊月新死者一枚，油一大升，煎之使烂，绞去滓，重煎成膏。涂冻疮及折破疮。

【注释】

［1］痫疾：根据文意，此处应为"疳疾"。

### 135. Mushu（Shu）［牡鼠（鼠），male mouse（mouse），Muroidea］

It is mainly used to treat the Gan disease[1] in children who have abdominal distention and rapacious appetite. Wrap it in the yellow mud, burn it, carefully pick out bones, use its meat to make thick soup with the ordinary cooking seasonings and eat it. Don't eat its bones because they can make people lose a lot of weight.

Decoct well one which dies in the twelfth lunar month with 1 Sheng of oil, wring out juice, filter it and decoct it again to make it into paste. The external application of the paste can be used to treat chilblain and the sore caused by the fracture damage.

【Note】

［1］ Gan disease：According to the first clause of the original text, here it should probably be "Gan disease" instead of "epilepsy". Chinese character "疳"（Gan disease）is similar to the character "痫"（epilepsy）in writing.

## 136. 蚌（蚌蛤） 大寒

主大热，解酒毒，止渴，去眼赤。动冷热气。

### 136. Bang（Bangge）［蚌（蚌蛤），clam, Anodonta Woodiana］ *severely cold*

It is mainly used to expel the severe heat, resolve the liquor toxin, relieve thirst and treat the red eyes. It can stir cold qi or heat qi.

## 137. 车 螯

（车螯）、蛦螯类，并不可多食之。

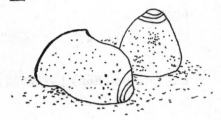

### 137. Che'ao［车螯，cheao clam，
### Meretrix Meretrix L.］

Some aquatic animals such as Che'ao［车螯，che'ao clam，Meretrix Meretrix L.］，Qingxie［青蟹，mud crab，Scylla Serrata］or Ribenxun［日本蟳，Japanese stone crab，Charybdis Japonica］can't be eaten excessively.

## 138. 蚶 温

（一）主心腹冷气，腰脊冷风。利五藏，建胃，令人能食。每食了，以饭压之。不尔令人口干。

（二）又云，温中，消食，起阳。味最重。出海中，壳如瓦屋。

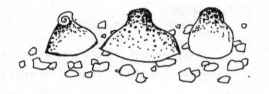

（三）又云，蚶：主心腹腰肾冷风，可火上暖之，令沸，空腹食十数个，以饮压之，大妙。

（四）又云，无毒。益血色。

（五）壳：烧，以米醋三度淬后埋，令坏。醋膏丸，治一切血气、冷气、症癖。

### 138. Han［蚶，arc clam，Arca Inflata Reeve］*warm*

It is mainly used to treat cold qi in the heart and abdomen and the disease caused by the invasion of cold wind in the waist and spine. It can regulate the five zang-organs, fortify the stomach and make people eat more. After eating it, eat some food to ease the side effect to avoid feeling dry mouth.

It can also be used to warm the middle, promote digestion and invigorate yang. It is the most effective in dealing with the problems mentioned above. It lives in the sea and its shell is similar to the corrugated tile.

It can also be mainly used to treat the disease caused by the invasion of cold wind in the heart, stomach, waist and kidney. Bake it with fire to make its juice in shell boil, eat more than ten of them on an empty stomach and eat some food to ease the side effect. It is especially effective.

It is non-toxic in property and can be used to make face ruddy and lustrous.

Burn its shell, dip it in Micu〔米醋, rice vinegar, Oryzae Acetum〕three times, bury it in earth to make it rot, and make paste or pills with vinegar to treat all kinds of insufficiency of qi and blood, cold qi, concretions and aggregations.

# 139. 蛏

（一）味甘,温,无毒。补虚,主冷利。煮食之,主妇人产后虚损。生海泥中,长二三寸,大如指,两头开。

（二）主胸中邪热、烦闷气。与服丹石人相宜。天行病后不可食,切忌之。

（三）又云,蛏:寒,主胸中烦闷邪气,止渴。须在饭食后,食之佳。

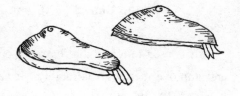

## 139. Cheng〔蛏, razor clam, Sinonovacula Constricta（Lamarck）〕

Sweet in taste and warm and non-toxic in property, it is used to supplement deficiency and treat the cold dysentery. Eating it after cooking is mainly used to treat women's postpartum vacuity detriment. It lives in the sea mud. It is 2 or 3 Cun long and as big as fingers. Both ends of its shell can open.

It is mainly used to eliminate the evil heat and vexation and oppression in the chest. It is suitable for the person who takes Danshi. Avoid eating it after recovering from the epidemic.

Cold in property, it is mainly used to eliminate the evil qi and vexation and oppression in the chest and relieve thirst. It is better to eat it after meal.

# 140. 淡 菜 温

（一）补五藏，理腰脚气，益阳事。能消食，除腹中冷气，消疹癖气。亦可烧，令汁沸出食之。多食令头闷、目暗，可微利即止。北人多不识，虽形状不典，而甚益人。

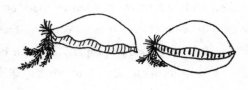

（二）又云，温，无毒。补虚劳损，产后血结，腹内冷痛。治症瘕，腰痛，润毛发，崩中带下。烧一顿令饱，大效。又名壳菜，常时频烧食即苦，不宜人。与少米先煮熟后，除肉内两边锁及毛了，再入萝蔔，或紫苏、或冬瓜皮同煮，即更妙。

## 140. Dancai［淡菜, mussel, Mytilus Edulis］*warm*

It is used to tonify the five zang-organs, treat the diseases in the waist and leg and improve men's sexual ability. It can be used to promote digestion, eliminate the cold qi in the abdomen and treat strings and aggregations. Stir-fry it to make its juice boil and overflow from its shell and eat it. Eating it excessively can cause dizziness and dim vision. It is suitable to eat a little and have a taste. Usually northerners do not know about it. Although it is not nice-looking, it can benefit people greatly.

Warm and non-toxic in property, it is used to supplement the deficiency due to the overstrain and vacuity detriment, treat the postpartum blood stasis, the cold and pain in the abdominal, abdominal mass, lumbago, profuse vaginal bleeding and women's leukorrheal disease and nourish the hair. It's quite effective in dealing with the problems mentioned above to cook it and eat one's fill. It is also called Qiaocai（壳菜）. It tastes bitter if cooked and eaten too often, thus it won't benefit people. After cooking with a small amount of rice, remove the tentacles and ligaments on both sides of its meat in shell, and add Luobo［萝卜, radish, Raphani Radix］, Zisu［紫苏, perilla, Perillae Folium, Caulis et Calyx］ or Dongguapi［冬瓜皮, wax gourd rind, Benincasae Exocarpium］ to cook again. It will be more effective.

## 141．虾 平

（一）无须及煮色白者,不可食。

（二）谨按:小者生水田及沟渠中,有小毒。小儿患赤白游肿[1],捣碎敷之。

（三）动风发疮疥。（勿作鲊食之）,鲊内者甚有毒尔。

【注释】

[1]赤白游肿:又名"赤白游风",是一种暂时性、局限性、无痛性的皮下或粘膜下水肿。西医称之为"血管性水肿",又称"巨大荨麻疹"。

### 141. Xia［虾, shrimp, Macrobrachium Nipponense］*mild*

It is inedible if it has no feeler or it turns white when cooked.

The following is supplemented by Zhang Ding: Slightly toxic in property, the small ones live in the paddy fields or ditches. Its crushed paste can be applied to the affected part to treat the red and white wandering wind[1] in children.

It can cause the wind qi and sores and scabies. Don't eat Zha made of it because it is severely toxic in property.

【Note】

[1] red and white wandering wind: A temporary, partial and painless subcutaneous or submucosal edema. In Western medicine it is also called angioneurotic edema or giant urticaria.

## 142．蛇蜕皮

主去邪,明目。治小儿一百二十种惊痫,寒热,肠痔[1],蛊毒,诸蜃恶疮,安胎。熬用之。

【注释】

[1]肠痔:病症名,肛门部痈疽。

### 142. Shetuipi［蛇蜕皮, snake slough, Serpentis Periostracum］

It is mainly used to eliminate the evil qi and improve vision. It is also used to treat one hundred and twenty kinds of fright epilepsies, deficiency cold or heat disease, intestinal hemorrhoid[1], parasitic toxin and all kinds of severe sores caused by the bite of ni worms and prevent miscarriage. Take it after decocting.

【Note】

[1] intestinal hemorrhoid: A disease, referring to the welling- and flat-abscesses in the anus.

## 143. 田 螺 大寒

汁饮疗热、醒酒、压丹石。不可常食。

### 143. Tianluo〔田螺, Chinese mystery snail, Cipangopaludina Chinensis Gray〕*severely cold*

Its juice is used to treat the heat disease, restore soberness and resolve the toxin of Danshi. Don't eat it regularly.

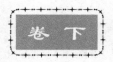

# Volume 3

## 144. 胡 麻[1]

（一）（胡麻）:润五藏,主火灼。山田种,为四棱[2]。土地有异,功力同。休粮人重之。填骨髓,补虚气。

（二）（青蘘）[3]:生杵汁,沐头发良。牛伤热亦灌之,立愈。

（三）（胡麻油）:主喑哑,涂之生毛发。

**【注释】**

［1］胡麻:一种油料作物,适宜在凉爽、湿润的气候生长,叶可食,有补益肝肾之功效。

［2］山田种,为四棱:胡麻节节结角,有一寸长。旧时认为胡麻随土地的肥瘠不同而结的角有四棱、八棱的区别。贫瘠土地出产的胡麻结角为四棱。

［3］青蘘(ráng):胡麻叶,味甘寒。

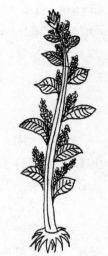

## 144. Huma[1]［胡麻, seed of oriental sesame, Semen Sesami Nigrum］

It can nourish the five zang-organs and mainly treat injury caused by fire inner heat. Its capsule pods have four sides[2] if planted in the barren soils of mountain areas. The clinic effects are the same though in different soil conditions. It is highly valued by the alchemists who practice inedia due to its effects of replenishing bones and marrows, supplementing deficiency and boosting qi.

The juice of Qingrang[3] has a good effect on washing hair. The same is true of the heat disease of cattle, taking some juice of it can help cattle recover very soon.

Huma［胡麻, seed of oriental sesame, Semen Sesami Nigrum］oil can treat the disease of dry and dumb throat, it is beneficial to the hair growth as well by applying it externally.

【Notes】

［1］Huma［胡麻, seed of oriental sesame, Semen Sesami Nigrum］: An oil crop growing in the cold and moist climate. Its leaves are edible with the effect of replenishing the liver and kidney.

［2］four sides: The length of the capsule pods of Huma is usually about 1 Cun. In the past, the capsule pods were thought to vary in different shapes with different soil conditions. Those growing in the barren lands have four sides while others in the fertile lands have eight.

［3］Qingrang: The leaves of Huma, sweet in taste and cold in property.

# 145. 白油麻

（一）大寒,无毒。治虚劳,滑肠胃,行风气,通血脉,去头浮风,润肌。食后生啖一合,终身不辍。与乳母食,其孩子永不病生。若客热,可作饮汁服之。停久者,发霍乱。又,生嚼敷小儿头上诸疮良。久食抽人肌肉。生则寒,炒则热。

（二）又,叶:捣和浆水,绞去滓,沐发,去风润发。

（三）其油:冷,常食所用也。无毒,发冷疾,滑骨髓,发藏腑渴,困脾藏,杀五黄,下三焦热毒气,通大小肠,治蛔心痛[1],敷一切疮疥癣,杀一切虫。取油一合,鸡子两颗,芒硝一两,搅服之,少时即泻,治热毒甚良。治饮食物,须逐日熬熟用,经宿即动气。有牙齿并脾胃疾人,切不可吃。陈者煎膏,生肌长肉,止痛,消痈肿,补皮裂。

【注释】

［1］蛔心痛:病名。因蛔虫移行乱窜引起的心腹中痛,时发时止。发病时疼痛难忍,伴有恶心呕吐,面色苍白,四肢冰冷。今见于胆管蛔虫症、蛔虫性肠梗阻、肠穿孔及腹膜炎等。

## 145. Baiyouma［白油麻, white oil sesame, Sesamum Indicum］

Severely cold and non-toxic in property, it can mainly treat the deficiency due to overstrain, nourish the intestines and stomach, move wind qi, disinhibit vessels, dispel the pathogenic wind in the head and moisten the skin. Taking 1 Ge of raw

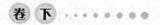

Baiyouma〔白油麻, white oil sesame, Sesamum Indicum〕after each meal can make people feel energetic. The mother in lactation, if taking it, will keep her baby healthy. The people suffering from the visiting heat can take the decoction of it. Do not take the long-stored decoction, or it may cause abrupt vomiting and diarrhea.

The chewed raw one has a good clinical effect on sores on the children's heads. Do not keep taking it for a long time, or it would consume muscles. The raw one is cold in property and the stir-baked is hot in property.

Its mashed leaves, mixing with the rice water and filtering with gauze, can be used to wash hair to dispel the head pathogenic wind and nourish hair.

Its oil, cold and non-toxic in property, is what we eat in daily life. It can cause the deficiency cold, exhaust bones and marrows and cause the consumptive thirst, vacuity detriment of visceras and stagnation of the spleen. It can treat five kinds of jaundice, eliminate heat toxin qi in the triple energizer, smooth the small and large intestines and treat the heartache caused by roundworms[1]. The external application of it can treat a variety of sores, scabies and tineas and kill parasites. Taking the mixture of 1 Ge of its oil, two eggs and 1 Liang of Mirabilite Glauber's Salt can cause diarrhea soon, which has a good effect on the heat toxin. The oil should be broiled well every day before cooking food; otherwise, it may stir qi easily. People with dental diseases and diseases in the spleen and stomach should not take it. Long-stored oil can be boiled into paste which can increase muscles, relieve pain, treat the abscess and heal the skin cracking.

**【Note】**

〔1〕heartache caused by roundworms: A heartache caused by the roundworms. The random moving of the roundworms in the abdomen causes the heartache on and off. It is characterized by the symptoms of pale face and cold limbs, vomiting and unbearable pain. Nowadays the diseases of Choledochyma, Ascaris Intestinal Obstruction and Intestinal Perforation and Peritonitis are common clinically.

## 146. 麻蕡[1]（麻子） 微寒

（一）治大小便不通，发落，破血，不饥，能寒。取汁煮粥，去五藏风，润肺，治关节不通，发落，通血脉，治气。

（二）青叶：甚长发。

（三）研麻子汁，沐发即生长。

（四）（消渴）：麻子一升捣，水三升，煮三、四沸，去滓冷服半升，日三，五日即愈。

（五）麻子一升，白羊脂七两，蜡五两，白蜜一合，和杵，蒸食之，不饥。

（六）《洞神经》[2] 又取大麻，日中服子末三升，东行茱萸根锉八升，渍之。平旦服之二升，至夜虫下。

（七）要见鬼者，取生麻子、菖蒲、鬼臼等分，杵为丸，弹子大。每朝向日服一丸。服满百日即见鬼也。

**【注释】**

［1］麻蕡(fén)：桑科植物大麻雌株的幼嫩果穗，味辛，性温，有毒，有祛风、止痛、镇痉之功效。

［2］《洞神经》：道藏佚书，系道家劾召鬼神之符书。

### 146. Mafen[1]（Mazi）［麻蕡（麻子），seed of hemp fimble, Semen Cannabis］ *slightly cold*

It can treat the urinary stoppage, constipation and alopecia, eliminate the blood stasis, make the stomach full and help resist the coldness. Making porridge with its juice can dispel the pathogenic wind in the five zang-organs, moisten the lung, disinhibit joints, treat alopecia, free the blood vessels and heal the qi disease.

Its leaves are of great benefit to hair growth.

Grinding it into juice and washing hair can benefit hair growth, too.

（Consumptive thirst）: Add 3 Sheng of water into 1 Sheng of pounded Mazi and boil them for 3 or 4 times, filter the residues and cool it. Taking half a Sheng of the decoction three times a day for five days in session can treat the consumptive thirst.

Pound 1 Sheng of it, 7 Liang of white goat fat, 5 Liang of wax and 1 Ge of white honey together and steam them. Taking the mixture of them can make the stomach full.

*Dong Shen Jing*[2] [《洞神经》, *Canon of Spirit Cultivation*] describes: Take 3 Sheng of the powder of seed of hemp fimble in the middle of the day. Grate 8 Sheng of the roots of Zhuyu [茱萸, evodia, Evodiae Fructus] which grow facing to the east and steep them into water for a night. Then drinking 2 Sheng of the mixture in the next morning may expel the parasites in the body.

Those who want to see ghosts may take one pill in the size of the marble made by the equal amounts of the raw seed of hemp fimble, Changpu [菖蒲, acorus, Acorus Calamus] and Guijiu [鬼臼, common dysosma, Rhizoma Dysosmae Versipellis] which are crashed together and face the sun every morning. After doing so for one hundred days, ghosts can be seen.

**【Notes】**

[1] Mafen: The young ears of the female cannabis in the family moraceae. It's pungent in taste, mild and toxic in property and has the effects of dispelling wind, relieving pain and relieving convulsion.

[2] *Dong Shen Jing*: An anonymous canon in Taoism which is used to summon ghosts.

# 147. 饴 糖

（一）饴糖：补虚，止渴，健脾胃气，去留血，补中。白者，以蔓菁[1]汁煮，顿服之。

（二）主吐血，健脾。凝强者为良。主打损瘀血，熬令焦，和酒服之，能下恶血。

（三）又，伤寒大毒嗽，于蔓菁、薤[2]汁中煮一沸，顿服之。

**【注释】**

[1] 蔓菁：见第 179 条"蔓菁"。

[2] 薤（xiè）：见第 197 条"薤"。

## 147. Yitang [饴糖, malt sugar, Maltosum]

It can tonify the deficiency and emaciation, allay the consumptive thirst, fortify the spleen and stomach, eliminate static blood and tonify the middle. Decoct the white one with the juice of Manjing[1] [蔓菁, turnip, Brassicae Rapae Tuber et Folium] and take the decoction in one go.

It can treat hematemesis and fortify the spleen. The more it solidifies, the better. It can mainly treat the static blood caused by knocks and falls. Boil it into the brown color and taking it with liquor can eliminate the malign blood.

Decoct it with the juice of Manjing [蔓菁, turnip, Brassicae Rapae Tuber et Folium] and Xie[2] [薤, Chinese chive, Allii Macrostemonis Bulbus] for boiling over one time, and take the decoction in one go, which can treat the cold and severe cough.

【Notes】
[1] Manjing: See Clause 179 "Manjing".
[2] Xie: See Clause 197 "Xie".

## 148. 大 豆 平

（一）主霍乱吐逆。

（二）微寒。主中风脚弱，产后诸疾。若和甘草煮汤饮之，去一切热毒气。

（三）善治风毒脚气，煮食之，主心痛，筋挛，膝痛，胀满。杀乌头、附子毒。

（四）大豆黄屑：忌猪肉。小儿不得与炒豆食之。若食了，忽食猪肉，必壅气致死，十有八九。十岁以上者不畏也。

（五）（大豆）卷：蘖长五分[1]者，破妇人恶血，良。

（六）大豆，寒。和饭捣涂一切毒肿。疗男女阴肿，以绵裹内之。杀诸药毒。

（又，生捣和饮，疗一切毒，服、涂之。）

（七）谨按：煮饮服之，去一切毒气，除胃中热痹[2]，伤中，淋露[3]，下淋血，散五藏结积内寒。和桑柴灰汁煮服，下水鼓腹胀。

（八）其豆黄：主湿痹，膝痛，五藏不足气，胃气结积，益气润肌肤。末之，收成炼猪膏为丸,服之能肥健人。

（九）又,卒失音,生大豆一升,青竹箅子四十九枚,长四寸,阔一分,和水煮熟,日夜二服,瘥。

（十）又,每食后,净磨拭,吞鸡子大,令人长生。初服时似身重,一年已后,便觉身轻。又益阳道。

【注释】

［1］分:古代的长度单位,唐代1分约合今制0.3厘米。

［2］热痹:病名,即热毒流注关节,或内有蕴热,复感风寒湿邪,与热相搏而致的痹症,又称"脉痹",可见关节红肿热痛、发热、烦闷、口渴等症。

［3］淋露:病名,可指女性月经淋沥不断或男女二便淋漓不尽、次数频繁之疾。

## 148. Dadou［大豆, soybean, Sojae Semen］ *mild*

It is mainly used to treat cholera and retching counterflow.

It is slightly cold in property. It can mainly treat stroke, weak feet and postpartum diseases. It can remove all kinds of heat toxin qi by decocting it with Gancao［甘草, licorice, Radix Glycyrrhea Praeparata］ and taking the decoction.

It is good at treating weak foot caused by the wind toxin. Taking the boiled ones can treat the heart pain, hypertonicity of the sinews, the pain of knees and distension and fullness and kill the toxin of Wutou［乌头, root of Szechwan aconita, Radix Aconiti］ and Fuzi［附子, aconite, Radix Aconiti Praeparata］.

The flake of black soys should be avoided to take with pork. Children should not take the fried beans. If children take pork immediately after taking fried beans, they will be most likely to die due to the congestion of qi dynamics. However, children aged more than ten are not afraid of that.

Soybeans with the sprout of 5 Fen[1] in length have a great effect of eliminating the malign blood in the woman's abdomen.

The soybean is cold in property. It can be pounded with cooked rice. Applying the mixture externally can treat all kinds of toxic swellings. It can treat the swelling and pain in the genitals of men and women by wrapping it with silk floss and applying it to the affected area. It can also kill the toxins of medicinals.

Pounding the raw ones and taking them with rice decoction can expel all kinds of toxic qi, the same is true of applying to the affected area externally.

The following is supplemented by Zhang Ding: Taking the decoction of it can expel all toxic qi, eliminate the heat impediment[2] in the stomach, treat the damage to the middle energizer, strangury diseases and lochia[3] and urine with blood and disperse the internal cold accumulated in the five zang-organs. Its decoction with the gray juice of mulberry twig can disperse the water drum distention and the abdominal distention.

The black soy is mainly used to treat the dampness impediment, the pain of knees, the insufficiency of the five zang-organs and qi stagnation in the stomach. It boosts qi and moistens the skin. Grind the black soy into powder and make it into medicinal pills with the extracted pork lard. The pills can fortify the body.

Boil 1 Sheng of raw soybeans and forty-nine bamboo chips with 4 Cun in length and 1 Fen in width with water. Taking it twice a day can cure the sudden loss of voice.

Rubbing an egg-sized handful of it and taking it after every meal can prolong life. People may feel heavy in the body at the very beginning of taking, but one year later, they may feel light. Long-term taking of it can invigorate Yang.

【Notes】

[1] Fen: A unit of length in ancient times. 1 Fen in the Tang Dynasty is roughly equivalent to 0.3 centimetre today.

[2] heat impediment: The name of a disease which is also known as a vessel impediment. The disease is caused by the confrontation of the heat toxin elements in joints with the invasion of wind, cold and dampness which can cause the pain and swelling of joints, fever, vexation, depression and thirst.

[3] strangury diseases and lochia: They refer to the persistent menstruation or dribbling after urination and defecation with high frequency.

## 149. 薏苡仁[1] 平

去干湿脚气,大验。

【注释】

[1] 薏苡仁:禾本科植物薏苡的干燥成熟种仁,味甘,有利水消肿、健脾去湿等功效。

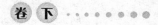

### 149. Yiyiren[1]〔薏苡仁，coix，Semen Coicis〕*mild*

It can treat the disease of beriberi caused by driness and dampness and has a good effect.

【Note】

〔1〕Yiyiren：The mature kernel of Coix which is a species of Genus Gramineae. It's sweet in taste and has the effects of disinhibiting water，dispersing swelling，fortifying the spleen and eliminating dampness.

# 150. 赤小豆

（一）和鲤鱼烂煮食之,甚治脚气及大腹水肿。别有诸治,具在鱼条中。散气,去关节烦热。令人心孔开,止小便数。菉、赤者并可食。

（二）止痢。暴痢后,气满不能食,煮一顿服之即愈。

（三）（毒肿）末赤小豆和鸡子白,薄之,立瘥。

（四）（风搔隐轸）[1]:煮赤小豆,取汁停冷洗之,不过三、四。

【注释】

〔1〕风搔隐轸:病名,相当于荨麻疹,是一种常见的皮肤病。症见患处皮肤出现大小不等之风团,奇痒难忍。多因阳气不足,外感风邪所致。

### 150. Chixiaodou〔赤小豆，rice bean，Semen Phaseoli〕

It can effectively treat weak foot and the enlarged abdomen with edema by boiling with carps and taking it. The other clinical effects are included in the entry of the Carp. Besides，it can disperse qi，eliminate the heat vexation in the joints，open the heart orifice and treat the frequent urination. The way of boiling with carps is true of Lvdou〔绿豆，mung bean，Vigna Radiata〕.

It can treat dysentery. Taking the boiled ones in one go can cure the inability to eat due to qi distention after the acute dysentery.

It can cure the toxic swelling instantly by applying its powder and egg white to the affected area.

It can cure urticarial[1] by using the cold soup of it to bathe the affected area three or four times.

【Note】

[1] urticarial：A common skin disease. It is characterized by the wind wheals in different sizes on the skin and the unbearable itch. It is mainly caused by the insufficiency of yang qi and the external contraction of wind evil.

## 151. 青小豆 寒

疗热中[1]，消渴，止痢，下胀满。

【注释】

[1] 热中：病症名，多指内热，是一类由于人体新陈代谢过于旺盛、产热过多所导致的疾病。

## 151. Qingxiaodou〔青小豆，mung bean，Vigna Radiata〕*cold*

It can treat the middle heat[1] and the consumptive thirst, check diarrhea and dysentery, and eliminate distention and fullness in the abdomen.

【Note】

[1] middle heat：A disease, usually referring to the internal heat. It is mainly caused by the vigorous metabolism and the excessive heat in the human body.

## 152. 酒

（一）味苦，主百邪毒，行百药。当酒卧，以扇扇，或中恶风。久饮伤神损寿。

（二）谨按：中恶痓忤，热暖姜酒一碗，服即止。

（三）又，通脉，养脾气，扶肝。陶隐居[1]云："大寒凝海，惟酒不冰"。量其热性故也。久服之，厚肠胃，化筋。初服之时，甚动气痢[2]。与百药相宜。祇服丹砂人饮之，即头痛吐热。

（四）又，服丹石人，胸背急闷热者，可以大豆一升，熬令汗出，簸去灰尘，投二升酒中。久时顿服之，少顷即汗出瘥。朝朝服之，甚去一切风。妇人产后诸风,亦可服之。

（五）又,熬鸡屎如豆淋酒[3]法作,名曰紫酒。卒不语、口偏者,服之甚效。

（六）昔有人常服春酒[4],令人肥白矣。

（七）紫酒:治角弓风。

（八）姜酒:主偏风中恶。

（九）桑椹酒:补五藏,明耳目。

（十）葱豉酒:解烦热,补虚劳。

（十一）蜜酒:疗风疹。

（十二）地黄、牛膝、虎骨、仙灵脾、通草、大豆、牛蒡、枸杞等,皆可和酿作酒,在别方。

（十三）蒲桃子酿酒,益气调中,耐饥强志,取藤汁酿酒亦佳。

（十四）狗肉汁酿酒,大补。

**【注释】**

[1] 陶隐居:即陶弘景(公元456—536年),字通明,南朝梁时丹阳秣陵(今江苏南京)人,号华阳隐居(自号华阳隐居),著名的医药家、炼丹家、文学家。

[2] 气痢:便痢赤白伴有肠鸣腹痛的痢疾,为中医病症名。

[3] 豆淋酒:豆淋酒用黑豆炒焦,以酒淋之;或大豆炒半熟,粗捣、筛、蒸,放入盆中,以酒淋之,去滓,主治破血祛风。

[4] 春酒:冬酿春熟之酒。

## 152. Jiu［酒, liquor, Vinum seu Spiritus］

It is bitter in taste. It can treat all kinds of evil qi and toxic qi, stimulate the efficacy of all kinds of drugs. When sleeping after drinking and fanning, it is likely to suffer from aversion to wind. Long-term drinking of it will damage the spirit and shorten life span.

The following is supplemented by Zhang Ding: It can treat the malignity stroke by taking one bowl of warm ginger liquor.

It can free vessels, nourish spleen qi and support the liver. Tao Yinju[1] said, "The severe cold can freeze the sea water but not the liquor." It's possible that the liquor is hot in property. Long-term drinking of it can strengthen the stomach and intestines, and free the sinews and bones. Drinking for the first time can often cause the qi dysentery[2]. It is compatible with all kinds of drugs. Those who only take Danshi will immediately suffer from headaches, vomiting and fever.

Those who take Danshi feeling the tightness, oppression and heat in their chests and backs, can decoct 1 Sheng of Dadou〔大豆, soybean, Sojae Semen〕until the steam is gone, remove the dust and put them into 2 Sheng of liquor, drink it at a time after a longer period of time. They will sweat after a while and get better. Drinking a little liquor every morning can dispel all kinds of wind evil. It can also dispel all kinds of women's postpartum wind evil.

The way of making the Doulin（豆淋）liquor[3] can be used to make Zijiu（purple liquor）which is made by drenching the decoction of droppings of chicken. It can effectively treat the sudden loss of voice and deviated mouth.

In the past, people often drank the spring liquor[4] which could make them plump and white.

The purple liquor can treat the arched-back rigidity.

The ginger liquor can treat the half-body wind paralysis and malignity stroke.

The mulberry wine can tonify the five-zang organs and improve hearing and vision.

The scallion and fermented soybean liquor can eliminate the vexing heat and tonify the deficiency due to overstrain.

The honey wine can treat the wind papules.

Dihuang〔地黄, rehmannia, Rehmanniae Radix〕, Niuxi〔牛膝, achyranthes, Achyranthis Bidentatae Radix〕, Hugu〔虎骨, tiger bone, Tigris Os〕, Xianlingpi〔仙灵脾, epimedium, Epimedii Herba〕, Tongcao〔通草, rice-paper plant pith, Tetrapanacis Medulla〕, Dadou〔大豆, soybean, Sojae Semen〕, Niubang〔牛蒡, arctium, Arctii Fructus〕, Gouqi〔枸杞, lycium, Lycii Fructus〕and so on can be added to Jiuniang〔酒酿, wine-fermented glutinous rice, Oryzae Glutinosae Semen cum Vino Fermentatum〕to make wines and the specific methods are in other formulas.

The grape seed wine can replenish qi, regulate the middle, make people tolerate hunger and strengthen memory. It is also effective to make wine with grape vine.

The liquor made with dog meat juice can greatly benefit the body.

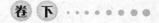

【Notes】

[1] Tao Yinju: He was also known as Tao Hongjing (456 – 536 A. D.), styling himself Tongming and having a literary name of Huayang Yinju, who was born in Moling, Danyang (now Nanjing, Jiangsu Province) in Liang Period of the Southern Dynasty. He was a famous physician, alchemist and writer.

[2] qi dysentery: It is the red and white dysentery. The patient who suffers from it has borborygmus and bellyache.

[3] Doulin liquor: A liquor made by stir-frying black beans to brown and drenching with wine or it can be made by stir-frying the soybeans until half done, crudely mashing, sieving, steaming, putting them into a basin, drenching with wine and filtering. It is mainly used to break blood and dispel wind.

[4] spring liquor: A liquor made in winter and drunk in spring.

# 153. 粟 米

陈者止痢,甚压丹石热。颗粒小者是。今人间多不识耳。其粱米粒粗大,随色别之。南方多畲田[1]种之。极易春,粒细,香美,少虚怯。祇为灰中种之,又不锄治故也。得北田种之,若不锄之,即草翳死;若锄之,即难春。都由土地使然耳。但取好地,肥瘦得所由,熟犁。又细锄,即得滑实。

【注释】

[1] 畲田:焚火种田,指以火耕的方式,用草木灰作基肥耕种的田地。

## 153. Sumi [粟米, foxtail millet seed, Semen Setariae Italicae]

The old one can treat dysentery and relieve the heat toxin of Danshi. Grains of Sumi [粟米, foxtail millet seed, Semen Setariae Italicae] are small while the grains of Liangmi [粱米, millet, Setariae Semen] are big in different colors. It is now difficult to tell the difference between them. It is extensively cultivated in She-Tian[1] (slash and burn fields) in the south, and the grains of it are mostly full, slender with savory smell and easy to pound. This is because of its growing in ash soil with no need to weed. Planted in the fields of the north, its seedlings will die due to the weed shade; if weeding, it will be difficult to pound the grains harvested from the seedlings. All of these are related to the different soils. To produce glossy and full grains, it is necessary to select a good field of proper fertility with adequate cultivation and careful weeding.

【Note】

[1] She-Tian: A way of cultivating the fields by fire. After burning the weeds in the fields, the plant ash can be used as the basic fertilizer to nourish the growing plants.

# 154. 秫 米[1]

（一）其性平。能杀疮疥毒热。拥五藏气，动风，不可常食。北人往往有种者，代米作酒耳。

（二）又，生捣和鸡子白，敷毒肿良。

（三）根：煮作汤，洗风。

（四）又：米一石，曲三升，和地黄一斤，茵陈蒿一斤，炙令黄，一依酿酒法。服之治筋骨挛急。

【注释】

[1] 秫米：在我国北方俗称"高粱米"，主要用于脾胃虚弱引起的夜寐不安，有和胃安眠之功效。

## 154. Shumi[1] [秫米, broomcorn millet, Panici Miliacei Semen]

It is mild in property. It can eliminate the heat toxin of sores and scabs. It may cause the congestion of qi movement in the five zang-organs and stir the wind qi, so it should not be taken often. The northern people plant it and often use it to substitute for rice to make liquor.

It can effectively treat the toxic swellings by applying the pounded raw one with egg white externally.

Decoct its root, and use the decoction to wash the affected area, which can eliminate the wind evil.

Stir-fry 1 Dan of it, 3 Sheng of distiller's yeast, 1 Jin of Dihuang [地黄, rehmannia, Rehmanniae Radix] and 1 Jin of Yinchenhao [茵陈蒿, virgate wormwood, Artemisiae Scopariae Herba] to yellow and brew them into liquor according to the routine brewing recipe. Taking the liquor can treat the inability of stretching the sinews and bones.

【Note】

[1] Shumi: It is also known as sorghum rice in the north of China. It mainly treats the restless sleep caused by the spleen-stomach vacuity and has the effects of harmonizing the stomach and quieting sleep.

# 155. 穬　麦[1]

主轻身,补中,不动疾。

【注释】

[1] 穬麦:大麦的一种,实熟时种子与稃壳分离,易脱落,种子供食用,亦作饲料,也称"裸大麦""青稞"。

## 155. Kuangmai[1]［穬麦, naked barley, Hordei Nudi Fructus］

It can relax the body and tonify the middle and does not cause diseases.

【Note】

[1] Kuangmai: A kind of barley. Its shell is easy to remove from the kernel when it is ripe. The kernel is both edible for people and cattle. It is also known as naked barley or highland barley.

# 156. 粳　米 平

(一)主益气,止烦(止)泄。其赤则粒大而香,不禁水停。其黄绿即实中。

(二)又,水渍有味,益人。都大新熟者,动气。经再年者,亦发病。江南贮仓人皆多收火稻。其火稻宜人,温中益气,补下元。烧之去芒。春春米食之,即不发病耳。

(三)仓粳米:炊作干饭食之,止痢。又补中益气,坚筋骨,通血脉,起阳道。

(四)北人炊之于瓮中,水浸令酸,食之暖五藏六腑之气。

(五)久陈者,蒸作饭,和醋封毒肿,立瘥。

(又,毒肿恶疮:久陈者,蒸作饭,和酢封肿上,立瘥。)

（六）又，研服之，去卒心痛。

（七）白粳米汁：主心痛，止渴，断热毒痢[1]。

（八）若常食干饭，令人热中，唇口干。不可和苍耳食之，令人卒心痛，即急烧仓米灰，和蜜浆服之，不尔即死。不可与马肉同食之，发痼疾。

（九）淮泗之间米多。京都、襄州土粳米亦香、坚实。又，诸处虽多，但充饥而已。

（十）性寒。拥诸经络气，使人四肢不收，昏昏饶睡。发风动气，不可多食。

【注释】

［1］热毒痢：病名，因骤受暑湿热毒所致的痢疾。

## 156. Jingmi［粳米，non-glutinous rice，Oryzae Semen］ *mild*

It can replenish qi, cease vexation and check diarrhea. The red-shelled grains are big and delicious, but they can't prevent water stagnation in the body. The yellow-green-shelled grains can fortify the spleen and stomach.

The one soaking in water is delicious and beneficial to people. Generally, the newly ripe one can cause the qi disease. The one stored for two years can also cause diseases. The southern people who store grains mostly collect rice growing in She-Tian. The rice growing in She-Tian can warm the middle, replenish qi and tonify the kidney qi. It is not easy to get diseases by burning away the awn tip of the shell and taking the pounded Jingmi［粳米，non-glutinous rice，Oryzae Semen］in spring.

Cooking the old Jingmi［粳米，non-glutinous rice，Oryzae Semen］and taking it can check dysentery. It can also tonify the middle, replenish qi, strengthen the sinews and bones, free the blood vessels and improve the sexual ability.

Northerners cook it in an earthen jar after soaking it in water and fermenting. Eating it can warm qi of the five zang-organs and six fu-organs.

Cook the rice stored for years and apply it to the toxic swelling with Cu［醋，vinegar，Acetum］and seal it, the swelling will be cured at once.

（To treat the toxic swelling and malign sores: Cook the rice stored for years and apply it to the toxic swelling with Cu［醋，vinegar，Acetum］and seal it, the swelling will be cured at once. )

Taking the ground powder of it can treat the sudden pain in the heart.

The soup of the white one can treat the pain in the heart, relieve thirst and eliminate the heat toxin dysentery[1].

The cooked rice should not be taken often, because it may cause the middle heat and the parched lips. It should not be taken with Cang'er [苍耳, xanthium herb, Xanthii Herba] because it may cause the sudden pain in the heart. Once that happens, take the burnt ash of the old rice with honey at once to save life. It should not be taken with the meat of Ma [马, horse, Equus Caballus] either, because it may cause the old intractable disease.

It is produced on a large scale in the basins of Huai River and Sishui River. The local one produced in Jingdu (now Xi'an, Shaanxi Province) and Xiangzhou (now Xiangyang, Hubei Province) is also delicious and has solid grains. It is also produced a lot in other places but only used to allay hunger.

Cold in property, it can block all kinds of channels qi, making people suffer from the weak limbs and somnolence. It can also cause the wind evil disease and the qi disease, so do not eat it too much.

【Note】

[1] heat toxin dysentery: A dysentery caused by the sudden heat, dampness and heat toxin.

# 157. 青粱米[1]

(一) 以纯苦酒一斗渍之,三日出,百蒸百暴,好裹藏之。远行一餐,十日不饥。重餐,四百九十日不饥。

(二) 又方,以米一斗,赤石脂三斤,合以水渍之,令足相淹。置于暖处二三日。上青白衣,捣为丸,如李大。日服三丸,不饥。

(三) 谨按:《灵宝五符经》中,白鲜米九蒸九暴,作辟谷粮。此文用青粱米,未见有别出处。其米微寒,常作饭食之,涩于黄,如白米,体性相似。

【注释】

[1] 青粱米:禾本科植物粱的一种,有健脾益气、涩精止泻等功效。按颜色的不同,粱可分为青粱米、白粱米、黄粱米等。

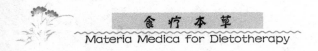

### 157. Qingliangmi[1] [青粱米, blue millet, Setariae Cyaneae Semen]

Steep it into 1 Dou of pure vinegar and take it out three days later. Steam and sun-dry it in turn for one hundred times. Then pack and store it. People who set out on a long journey can take it for one meal, and then they will be full for ten days. If taking another meal more, they will be full for four hundred and ninety days.

Submerge 1 Dou of it and 3 Jin of Chishizhi [赤石脂, halloysite, Halloysitum Rubrum] and put the mixture in warm place for two or three days in order to make it covered by a layer of blue and white mycelia. After that, pound it into pills in the size of plums. Taking three pills a day can make the stomach full.

The following is supplemented by Zhang Ding: It is recorded in *Ling Bao Wu Fu Jing* [《灵宝五符经》, *The Canon of Spirit Preservation and Five Incantations*] that the fresh rice, steamed and sun-dried nine times, can be used as the food in inedia. Here it mentions Qingliangmi [青粱米, blue millet, Setariae Cyaneae Semen], the recipe cannot be found from the other books. It is slightly cold in property and is usually cooked as meal. Its taste is more astringent than that of the yellow millet, similar to that of the white one. The shape and effect are similar to those of the white millet.

【Note】

[1] Qingliangmi: One kind of millet which is the gramineous plant. It has the effects of fortifying the spleen, boosting qi, astringing essence and checking diarrhea. Due to the different colors, the millet can be classified into blue millet, white millet and yellow millet.

### 158. 白粱米[1]

（一）患胃虚并呕吐食及水者，用米汁二合，生姜汁一合，和服之。

（二）性微寒。除胸膈中客热，移易五藏气，续筋骨。此北人长食者是，亦堪作粉。

【注释】

[1] 白粱米：禾本科植物粱的一种，味甘，性微寒，有益气、和中、除烦、止渴之功效。按颜色的不同，粱可分为青粱米、白粱米、黄粱米等。

## 158. Bailiangmi[1] [白粱米, white millet, Setariae Albae Semen]

Those who have the disease of stomach deficiency and vomiting food and water can take the mixture of 2 Ge of its soup and 1 Ge of fresh ginger juice.

It is slightly cold in property and can eliminate the visiting heat in the chest and diaphragm, regulate the qi movement of the five zang-organs and join the sinews and bones. It is the main food for northerners and can be taken in the form of flour.

【Note】

[1] Bailiangmi: One kind of millet which is the gramineous plant. It is sweet in taste and slightly cold in property. It has the effects of boosting qi, harmonizing the middle, eliminating vexation and quenching thirst. Due to the different colors, the millet can be classified into blue millet, white millet and yellow millet.

## 159. 黍 米[1] 寒

（一）患鳖瘕[2]者,以新熟赤黍米,淘取泔汁,生服一升,不过二三度愈。

（二）谨按:性寒,有少毒。不堪久服,昏五藏,令人好睡。仙家重此。作酒最胜余米。

（三）又,烧为灰,和油涂杖疮,不作瘢,止痛。

（四）不得与小儿食之,令儿不能行。若与小猫、犬食之,其脚便蹋曲,行不正。缓人筋骨,绝血脉。

（五）和葵菜食之,成痼疾。于黍米中藏干脯通。《食禁》云:牛肉不得和黍米、白酒食之,必生寸白虫。

（六）黍之茎穗:人家用作提拂,以将扫地。食苦瓠毒,煮汁饮之即止。

（七）又,破提扫煮取汁,浴之去浮肿。

（八）又,和小豆煮汁,服之下小便。

【注释】

[1] 黍米:一年生草本植物,其颗粒大于小米,呈金黄色,黏度很大,具有滋补肾阴、健脾活血等功效。

[2] 鳖瘕:病症名,指腹中如鳖状的瘕结,多由脾胃虚弱、受冷饮食不消化所致。

## 159. Shumi[1] [黍米, broomcorn millet, Panici Miliacei] *cold*

Use water to wash the newly-harvested Shumi [黍米, broomcorn millet, Panici Miliacei] with the red shells. Taking the washing water of it two or three times can cure the disease of turtle movable abdominal mass[2].

The following is supplemented by Zhang Ding: It is cold and slightly toxic in property. It should not be taken for a long time, because it may cause the confusion of the five zang-organs and somnolence. Those who pursue immortality value it more. It is better than the other kinds of millets to make liquor.

The burnt-ash of it, mixed with oil, can be applied externally to the wound caused by the rod punishment to avoid limp and relieve the pain.

Children should not take it, because it may make their legs too weak to walk. Little cats and dogs should not take it either, because it may make their legs too distorted to walk straight. It may cause the weak and slack sinews and bones and exhaust the blood vessels.

Taking it with Kuicai [葵菜, mallow, Malva verticillata] can cause the intractable diseases. The dried meat can be stored in it. *Shi Jin* [《食禁》, *The Dietary Contraindication*] records that beef should not be taken with it and Baijiu [白酒, white liquor, Granorum Spiritus Incolor], because this mixture may breed tapeworms.

The stems and ears of it are usually made into brooms to sweep. Its decoction can resolve the toxin caused by eating Kuhu [苦瓠, bitter calabash, Lagenariae Gourdae].

Using the decoction of the old brooms made by the stems and ears of it to shower can disperse the puffy swelling.

The decoction of it with Xiaodou [小豆, black gram, Phaseoli Mungo Semen] can disinhibit the urine.

【Notes】

[1] Shumi: An annual plant. Its grains are bigger than those of Xiaomi [小米, millet, Setariae Semen] with golden color and great stickiness. It has the effects of enriching yin, supplementing the kidney, fortifying the spleen and quickening the

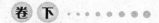

blood.

[2] turtle movable abdominal mass: A disease. It refers to the abdominal mass in the size of a turtle and is mainly caused by the spleen-stomach deficiency and dietary indigestion due to the coldness.

## 160. 稷[1]

（一）益气,治诸热,补不足。

（二）山东多食。服丹石人发热,食之热消也。发三十六种冷病气。八谷之中,最为下苗。黍乃作酒,此乃作饭,用之殊途。

（三）不与瓠子同食,令冷病发。发即黍酿汁,饮之即差。

【注释】

[1] 稷:禾本科植物,味甘,无毒,有和中益气、凉血解暑之功效。与黍同类,黏者为黍,不黏者为稷。

## 160. Ji[1] [稷, non-glutinous broomcorn millet, Panici Non-Glutinosi Semen]

It can replenish qi, treat all kinds of heat diseases and tonify insufficiency.

It is the main food for people living in the north of Taihang Mountain. Taking it can eliminate Danshi heat in the body. It causes thirty-six kinds of deficiency cold. Among the eight cereals, it ranks the lowest. Shu [黍, broomcorn millet, Panici Miliacei] is used to make liquor while it is used to make food, those two varying in application.

It should not be taken with Huzi [瓠子, sweet gourd, Lagenariae Clavatae Fructus], for it may cause the deficiency cold. Once that happens, people can take the sour broomcorn millet water to treat it.

【Note】

[1] Ji: A gramineous plant. It's sweet in taste and non-toxic in property and has the effects of harmonizing the middle, replenishing qi, cooling the blood and clearing the summer heat. It is classified as the same group as Shu [黍, broomcorn millet, Panici Miliacei]. The difference between these two is that Shu [黍, broomcorn millet, Panici Miliacei] has the nature of stickiness while it does not.

# 161. 小 麦<sup>[1]</sup> 平

（一）养肝气，煮饮服之良。服之止渴。

（二）又云：面有热毒者，为多是陈黦之色。

（三）又，为磨中石末在内，所以有毒，但杵食之即良。

（四）又宜作粉食之，补中益气，和五藏，调经络，续气脉。

（五）又，炒粉一合，和服断下痢。

（六）又，性主伤折，和醋蒸之，裹所伤处便定。重者，再蒸裹之，甚良。

【注释】

[1] 小麦：世界各地广泛种植的禾本科植物，富含淀粉、蛋白质、脂肪、矿物质、钙、铁等，具有解热和中、消渴止烦等功效。

# 161. Xiaomai<sup>[1]</sup>〔小麦，wheat，Tritici Semen〕 *mild*

It can nourish the liver qi and has a good effect by taking its boiled soup. It can quench thirst.

The old flour of yellow and black color usually has the heat toxin.

The stone-ground flour has stone powder in it, so it has the toxin, while the pestle-ground flour does not have the toxin, so it is safe to eat.

It is suitable to make into flour. It can tonify the middle, replenish qi, harmonize the five zang-organs, regulate collaterals, and continue qi and vessels.

Taking 1 Ge of its fried flour with water can check dysentery.

Steaming it with vinegar, wrapping and applying it to the injuries can treat the injured and broken sinews and bones. Repeating the procedure can treat the severe injuries more effectively.

【Note】

[1] Xiaomai: A gramineous plant widespreadly cultivated around the world. It's rich in starch, protein, fat, minerals, calcium and iron and has effects of resolving heat, harmonizing the middle, dispersing thirst and ceasing vexation.

## 162. 大 麦

（一）久食之，头发不白。和针沙、没石子[1]等染发黑色。

（二）暴食之，（亦稍似）令脚弱，为（下气及）腰肾间气故也。久服即好，甚宜人。

（三）熟即益人，带生即冷，损人。

【注释】

[1] 没石子：昆虫没食子蜂的幼虫寄生于植物没食子树幼枝上所产生的虫瘿，具有固气、涩精、敛肺、止血等功效。古人常将针沙与没石子混合，用于染发。

## 162. Damai［大麦，barley，Hordei Fructus］

Taking it for a long time can keep the hair black. Its flour with steel filings and Moshizi[1]［没石子，Aleppo gall，Galla Halepensis］can dye the hair black.

The sudden taking of it may result in slightly weak legs and feet, because it can precipitate qi and consume yang qi of the kidney and lumbus, while taking it for a along time can get better, because it can greatly benefit health.

The well-cooked one can do good to people whereas the half-cooked one, cold in property, can harm people.

【Note】

[1] Moshizi：The gall insect produced by the larva of gall wasps when living on the young shoots of the Quercus infectoria Oliv. It has the effects of securing qi, astringing essence, constraining the lung and stanching bleeding. The ancient people usually mixed the steel filings and Moshizi together to dye hair.

## 163. 曲[1]

（一）味甘，大暖。疗藏腑中风气，调中下气，开胃消宿食。主霍乱，心膈气，痰逆。除烦，破症结及补虚，去冷气，除肠胃中塞、不下食。令人有颜色。六月作者良,陈久者入药。用之当炒令香。

(二)六畜食米胀欲死者,煮曲汁灌之,立消。落胎,并下鬼胎。

(三)又,神曲[2],使[3],无毒。能化水谷,宿食,症气。健脾暖胃。

【注释】

[1]曲:在酿酒和制酱过程中一种用于发酵的物质,具有祛风寒、助消化等功效。

[2]神曲:主治食积、泻痢,也可用以酿酒。

[3]使:即中医药方中的使药,一是指引经药(即引方中诸药到达病所的药物),二是指调和药(即具有调和诸药作用的药物)。

## 163. Qu[1][曲, yeast, Materia Medica Qu]

It is sweet in taste and severely hot in property. It can treat the wind evil in the zang-fu organs, regulate the middle, precipitate qi, increase the appetite and disperse the accumulated food. It can also treat the cholera, qi stagnation in the heart, the copious phlegm and qi counterflow, eliminate vexation, disperse concretions and binds, supplement deficiency, expel cold qi, eliminate the blockage of the stomach and intestines, treat the inability to get food down and make the complexion good. Those made in the sixth lunar month have good quality. Those stored for a long time can be used as medicinals. It should be fried when used as medicinals.

If the six domestic animals are going to die of the abdominal distention due to the excessive intake of millet, taking its decoction can eliminate the distention instantly. It can abort fetus and even eliminate phantom pregnancy.

Shenqu[2], non-toxic in property, can be used as a channel conductor[3]. It can transform water and cereals, eliminate the accumulated food, disperse qi stagnation of the concretions and binds in the abdomen, fortify the spleen and warm the stomach.

【Notes】

[1] Qu: Something that causes the fermentation in the process of making liquor and sauce. It has the effects of dispersing wind cold and aiding digestion.

[2] Shenqu: It can treat food accumulation, diarrhea and dysentery. It can also

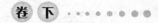

be used to make liquor.

[3] channel conductor: In Traditional Chinese Medicine prescriptions, there are two kinds of medicinals that can be used as a channel conductor. The first one refers to the channel ushering drugs that can usher the other drugs in the prescription to the infected area. The second refers to the harmonizing drugs that can harmonize the effects of the other drugs in the prescription.

# 164. 荞 麦 <sub>寒</sub>

（一）难消,动热风。不宜多食。

（二）虽动诸病,犹压丹石。能练五藏滓秽,续精神。其叶可煮作菜食,甚利耳目,下气。其制为灰,洗六畜疮疥及马扫蹄至神。

（三）味甘平,寒,无毒。实肠胃,益气力,久食动风,令人头眩。和猪肉食之,患热风,脱人眉须。虽动诸病,犹挫丹石。能铄五藏滓秽,续精神。作饭与丹石人食之,良。其饭法:可蒸使气馏,于烈日中暴,令口开,使舂取人作饭。叶作茹食之,下气,利耳目。多食即微泄。烧其穰作灰,淋洗六畜疮,并驴马躁蹄。

## 164. Qiaomai [荞麦, buckwheat, Fagopyri Semen] *cold*

It is hard to digest and can cause the wind heat, so it cannot be taken too much.

Even though it may cause all kinds of diseases, it can inhibit Danshi toxin. It can eliminate dregs and waste in the five zang-organs and boost spirit. Its leaves can be boiled as dishes which can improve sight and hearing and precipitate qi. It can effectively treat the sores on the six domestic animals and the sores on the horse's hoofs by using the ash of its stems with water to wash the affected area.

It is sweet in taste and mild, cold and non-toxic in property. It can fortify the stomach and intestines, replenish qi and energy. But the frequent taking of it can cause wind qi and dizzy head. Taking it with pork can cause wind heat and shed eyebrows and beard. Even though it may cause all kinds of diseases, it can inhibit Danshi toxin. It can eliminate dregs and waste in the five zang-organs and boost spirit. Those who take Danshi are especially suitable to take it cooked. Here is the recipe to cook it: Steam it until the vapor goes upwards and sun-burn it in the scorching sunlight, which can make its shells cracked. Thus its kernels can be pounded out and cooked. Its leaves can be boiled as dishes which can improve sight and hearing and precipitate qi. It can cause the slight diarrhea if taken too much. It can effectively treat the sores on the six domestic animals and the sores on the horse's hoofs by using the ash of its stems with water to wash the affected area.

## 165. 藊豆（扁豆） <sub>微寒</sub>

（一）主呕逆,久食头不白。患冷气人勿食。

（二）疗霍乱吐痢不止,末和醋服之,下气。

（三）其叶治瘕[1],和醋煮。理转筋,叶汁醋服效。

（四）又,吐痢后转筋,生捣叶一把,以少酢浸,取汁服之,立瘥。

（五）其豆如菉豆,饼食亦可。

【注释】

[1] 瘕:病症名,即瘕病,症见因寒温不适导致的饮食不消,与藏气相搏,积在腹内,结块瘕痛,随气移动。

## 165. Biandou [藊豆（扁豆）, lablab, Lablab Semen Album] *slightly cold*

It can treat the retching counterflow. Taking it for a long time can maintain the hair black. Those who suffer from cold qi should not take it.

It can treat the vomiting and diarrhea caused by cholera. Taking its powder with vinegar can precipitate qi.

The leaves can treat the movable abdominal mass[1] by taking the decoction of them with vinegar. The leaves can also treat cramp by taking their juice with vinegar.

Pound a handful of fresh leaves of it and use a small amount of vinegar to macerate them. Taking their juice can treat the cramp caused by the treatment of vomiting and diarrhea.

It is in the size of Lüdou [菉豆, mung bean, Phaseoli Radiati Semen] and can be cooked as cakes.

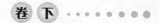

【Note】

[1] movable abdominal mass: A disease characterized by the non-digestion of food due to the coldness fighting with zang qi, accumulating in the abdomen, forming lumps and moving with qi.

## 166. 豉[1]

（一）能治久盗汗患者,以二升微炒令香,清酒三三升渍。满三日取汁,冷暖任人服之,不瘥,更作三两剂即止。

（二）陕府豉汁甚胜于常豉。以大豆为黄蒸,每一斗加盐四升,椒四两,春三日,夏二日,冬五日即成。半熟,加生姜五两,既洁且精,胜埋于马粪中。黄蒸,以好豉心代之。

【注释】

[1] 豉:一种用熟的黄豆或黑豆经发酵后制成的食品,可以调味,也可入药。

### 166. Chi[1] [豉, fermented soybean, Semen Sojae Preparatum]

It can treat the long-term night sweat. Stir-fry 2 Sheng of it with the low flame until smelling fragrant, add 3 Sheng of clear liquor to macerate it and extract the juice three days later. Patients can choose to take it hot or cold at their own will. With no effect, patients can take two or three more doses made by the same formula. The night sweat will be cured.

The fermented soybean sauce in Shaanxi Province is much better than that in other places, which is made by the yeast steamed from the soybeans according to the formula that 1 Dou of soybeans are with 4 Sheng of salt and 4 Liang of zanthoxylum. The making process will take three days in spring, two days in summer and five days in winter to complete. In the middle of fermentation, the addition of 5 Liang of fresh ginger may guarantee the cleanness and good quality, which makes this kind of sauce better than the kind fermented in horseshit. The best Chixin must be used in the process of soaking, steaming and fermenting.

【Note】

[1] Chi: A food made by the fermentation of the steamed soybeans or black

soybeans. It can be used both as seasoning and as drug.

# 167. 菉豆[1]（绿豆） 平

（一）诸食法,作饼炙食之佳。

（二）谨按:补益,和五藏,安精神,行十二经脉。此最为良。今人食,皆挞去皮,即有少拥气。若愈病,须和皮,故不可去。

（三）又,研汁煮饮服之,治消渴。

（四）又,去浮风,益气力,润皮肉。可长食之。

【注释】

[1] 菉豆:豆科植物绿豆,味甘,性寒,有清凉解毒、利尿明目等功效。

## 167. Lüdou (Lüdou)[1][菉豆（绿豆）, mung bean, Phaseoli Radiati Semen] *mild*

Among many recipes of cooking it, the best way is to make it into cakes and fry it.

The following is supplemented by Zhang Ding：It has good effects to tonify the body, harmonize the five zang-organs, tranquilize mind and move the twelve meridians. Nowadays its seed-coats are usually removed by beating before taking, which may to some extent block the qi dynamic. It can effectively treat diseases with the seed-coats on.

It can treat the consumptive thirst by taking its decoction.

It can also disperse the superficial wind, replenish qi and energy and moisten the skin and muscles. So it can be taken for a long term.

【Note】

[1] Lüdou (Lüdou)：It is a species of Genus Leguminosae, sweet in taste and cold in property, which has the effects of cooling, removing toxin, disinhibiting urine and brightening the eyes.

# 168. 白 豆[1]

平,无毒。补五藏,益中,助十二经脉,调中,暖肠胃。叶:利五藏,下气。嫩者可作菜食。生食之亦妙,可常食。

【注释】

[1] 白豆:豆科植物菜豆的种子,具有补肾健脾、生精止渴等功效。

## 168. Baidou[1][白豆, kidney bean, Phaseoli Vulgaris Semen]

It is mild and non-toxic in property. It can tonify the five zang-organs, replenish the spleen and the stomach, aid the twelve meridians, regulate the middle and warm the stomach and intestines. Its leaves can replenish the five zang-organs and precipitate qi. The young leaves can be cooked as dishes, which can also be taken raw often.

【Note】

[1] Baidou: The kernel of the asparagus bean which is a species of Genus Leguminosae. It has the effects of tonifying the kidney, fortifying the spleen, engendering essence and quenching thirst.

## 169. 醋(酢酒)

(一)多食损人胃。消诸毒气,煞邪毒。能治妇人产后血气运[1]:取美清醋,热煎,稍稍含之即愈。

(二)又,人口有疮,以黄蘖皮醋渍,含之即愈。

(三)又,牛马疫病,和灌之。

(四)服诸药,不可多食。不可与蛤肉同食,相反。

(五)又,江外人多为米醋,北人多为糟醋。发诸药,不可同食。

(六)(酢)研青木香服之,止卒心痛、血气等。

(七)又,大黄涂肿,米醋飞丹用之。

(八)治痃癖[2],醋煎大黄,生者甚效。

(九)用米醋佳,小麦醋不及。糟多妨忌,大麦醋,微寒。余如小麦(醋)也。

(十)气滞风壅,手臂、脚膝痛:炒醋糟裹之,三两易,当瘥。人食多,损腰肌藏。

【注释】

[1] 产后血气运:产后血晕,病名,多因产后血虚气脱或血瘀气逆所致。

[2] 痃癖:痃癖气,病名,脐腹偏侧或胁肋部时有筋脉攻撑急痛的病症。

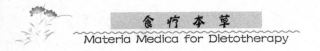

## 169. Cu（Zhajiu）［醋(酢酒)，vinegar，Acetum］

It can damage the stomach if taken too much. It can resolve all kinds of toxic qi and expel the evil toxin. It can also treat women's postpartum blood dizziness[1] by decocting the good one till it is hot and containing it in the mouth.

It can treat the mouth sore by containing Huangbo［黄蘗，phellodendron，Phellodendri Cortex］soaked in it in the mouth.

It can treat the infectious diseases of Ma［马，horse，Equus Caballus］or Niu［牛，cattle，Bovidae］by making the animal drink it.

It should not be taken too much when drugs are taken. It should not be taken with Bangge［蚌蛤，clam，Anodonta Woodiana］，because these two clash with each other.

Southerners often use rice to make it while northerners often use Jiuzao［酒糟，liquor dregs，Vini Residuum］to make it. It should not be taken with drugs because it can cause the toxicity of all kinds of drugs.

It can treat the sudden pain in the heart and all kinds of diseases caused by the insufficient blood qi by grinding Qingmuxiang［青木香，aristolochia root，Aristolochiae Radix］soaked in it into powder and taking the powder.

Water grind Dahuang［大黄，rhubarb，Rhei Radix et Rhizoma］with it into powder and make elixirs with the powder. They can treat the swollen sore by the external application.

The decoction of Dahuang［大黄，rhubarb，Rhei Radix et Rhizoma］with it can treat the paraumbilical and hypochondriac aggregation[2]. The decoction will have great effects with Shengdahuang［生大黄，raw rhubarb，Rhei Radix et Rhizoma Crudi］.

For the medical purpose, that made of rice is better than that made of Xiaomai［小麦，wheat，Tritici Semen］. There are some contraindications in using that made of Jiuzao［酒糟，liquor dregs，Vini Residuum］. Though that made of Damai［大麦，barley，Hordei Fructus］is slightly cold in property, it is the same as that made of Xiaomai［小麦，wheat，Tritici Semen］in other respects.

To treat the qi stagnation, the wind evil obstruction and pain in the arms, feet

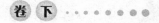

and knees：Stir-fry Cuzao〔醋糟, vinegar residue, Aceti Residuum〕to make it hot and apply it to the affected area after wrapping. After two or three times the disease mentioned above will be cured. Drinking too much of it will damage essence qi in the waist.

【Notes】

〔1〕postpartum blood dizziness：It is a disease caused by the postpartum blood deficiency and qi desertion or blood stasis and qi counterflow.

〔2〕paraumbilical and hypochondriac aggregation：A disease. It refers to the sharp pain caused by the attack of the tendons and muscles at the side of the umbilicus or in the hypochondriac region.

## 170. 糯 米[1] 寒

（一）使人多睡。发风,动气,不可多食。

（二）又,霍乱后吐逆不止,清水研一碗,饮之即止。

【注释】

〔1〕糯米:又被称为"江米",是家常食用粮食之一,具有补中益气、健胃养脾等功效。

## 170. Nuomi[1]〔糯米, glutinous rice, Oryzae Glutinosae Semen〕*cold*

It can cause somnolence, wind evil and qi disease. So it should not be taken too much.

It can check the incessant retching counterflow due to cholera by grinding it with clean water and taking one bowl of the mixture.

【Note】

〔1〕Nuomi：One of the major grains in people's daily life. It is also known as Jiangmi and has the effects of tonifying the middle, replenishing qi, fortifying the stomach and nourishing the spleen.

## 171. 酱

（一）主火毒,杀百药。发小儿无辜[1]。

（二）小麦酱：不如豆。

（三）又，榆仁酱：亦辛美，杀诸虫，利大小便，心腹恶气。不宜多食。

（四）又，芜荑酱：功力强于榆仁酱。多食落发。

【注释】

［1］无辜：小儿疳类疾病，症见小儿因慢性营养不良而导致的身体虚弱羸瘦。

## 171. Jiang［酱，paste，Pasta］

It can treat the fire toxin, lessen the efficacy of all kinds of drugs and may make children suffer from Wugu disease[1].

Wheat sauce is not better than bean paste.

Yurenjiang［榆仁酱，dwarf elm fruit jam, Ulmi Pumilae Fructus Praeparatio］, pungent, fragrant and delicious in taste, can kill all kinds of parasites, disinhibit the urine and stool and disperse the malign qi in the heart and abdomen. But it cannot be taken too much.

The drug effect of Wuyijiang［芜荑酱，elm fruit liquid, Ulmi Fructus Praeparatio Liquida］is more powerful than that of Yurenjiang［榆仁酱，dwarf elm fruit jam, Ulmi Pumilae Fructus Praeparatio］. Taking too much of it can cause hair loss.

【Note】

［1］Wugu disease：A disease of infantile malnutrition. It is characterized by infantile weakness and thinness due to malnutrition.

## 172. 葵（冬葵）冷

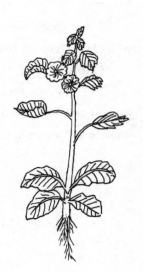

（一）主疳疮生身面上、汁黄者：可取根作灰，和猪脂涂之。

（二）其性冷，若热食之，亦令人热闷。甚动风气。久服丹石人时吃一顿，佳也。

（三）冬月，葵葅汁。服丹石人发动，舌干咳嗽，每食后饮一盏，便卧少时。

（四）其子，患疮者吞一粒，便作头。

（五）主患肿未得头破者，三日后，取葵子二百粒，吞之，当日疮头开。

（六）女人产时，可煮，顿服之佳。若生时困闷，以子一合，水二升，煮取半升，去滓顿服之，少时便产。

（又，凡有难产，若生未得者，取一合捣破，以水二升，煮取一升已下，只可半升，去滓顿服之，则小便与儿便出。切须在意，勿上厕。昔有人如此，立扑儿入厕中。）

（七）又，（苗叶）细锉，以水煎服一盏食之，能滑小肠。

（八）（叶）：女人产时，煮一顿食，令儿易出。

（九）（根）：天行病后，食一顿，便失目。

（十）吞钱不出，（根）煮汁，冷饮之，即出。

（十一）无蒜勿食。四季月食生葵，令饮食不消化，发宿疾。

（十二）又，霜葵生食，动五种留饮[1]。黄葵尤忌。

**【注释】**

［1］留饮：病症名，是指水饮蓄留体内，聚于胸膈胁腹或四肢关节，影响有关脏腑组织功能。

## 172. Kui（Dongkui）［葵（冬葵），mallow，Malva Crispa Linn.］ *cold*

It can treat the Gan sore with yellow pus on the body and face by burning its root into ash and applying it to the sore with Zhuzhi［猪脂，pork lard，Suis Adeps］.

It is cold in property，but it will cause heat and oppression if taken warm. It is very likely to cause wind qi. It is good for people who take Danshi for a long time to eat it occasionally.

The juice of Dongkui［冬葵，mallow，Malva Crispa Linn.］made in winter can treat the dry tongue and cough due to the medicinal toxicity of Danshi by taking 1 Zhan of it and lying down for a while.

People suffering from swollen sore can swallow a seed，and the sore will form a pus head.

It can treat the non-eruption of the pus head after the patient suffers from swollen sore for three days. The patient can take 200 seeds，and then the pus head will erupt in the same day.

The woman in labor can drink the boiled seed juice at a time, and it is very effective. If the woman in labor feels oppressed and difficult to deliver, she can decoct 1 Ge of the seeds with 2 Sheng of water into half a Sheng of decoction, filter the decoction, get rid of the dregs and take it at a time. After a while the baby will be delivered.

(If the woman in labor has difficulty in delivery or the baby cannot be completely delivered, she can decoct 1 Ge of the mashed seeds with 2 Sheng of water into less than 1 Sheng of decoction, preferably half a Sheng, filter the decoction and take it at a time. Then the baby will be discharged with urine. Don't go to the toilet at this time. In the past, the woman in labor went to the toilet and the baby fell into the toilet.)

It can disinhibit the small intestine by taking 1 Zhan of the decoction of the chopped thin leaves.

The woman in labor can eat the boiled leaves at a time to make it easy to give birth.

The person who has contracted an epidemic disease will lose the sight if he or she eats the root.

If a person swallows a coin and the coin can't be excreted, he can drink the cool decoction of the root and the coin will be excreted.

It should not be taken without Dasuan〔大蒜, garlic, Allii Sativi Bulbus〕. The uncooked Dongkui〔冬葵, mallow, Malva Crispa Linn.〕should not be taken in the third, sixth, ninth and twelfth lunar month, because it may cause indigestion and recurrence of the old disease.

The uncooked Dongkui〔冬葵, mallow, Malva Crispa Linn.〕should not be taken after the frost either, because it may cause five kinds of prolonged fluid retention diseases[1]. Huangkui〔黄葵, abelmosk, Abelmoschi Moschati Radix seu Folium〕is particularly forbidden to eat.

【Note】

[1] prolonged fluid retention disease: A disease. It refers to the retention of fluid in the body, gathering in the flank of the chest or the joints of limbs, affecting the function of the zang-fu organs.

# 173. 苋（苋菜）

（一）补气，除热。其子明目。九月霜后采之。

（二）叶：食亦动气，令人烦闷，冷中损腹。

（三）不可与鳖肉同食，生鳖症[1]。又取鳖甲如豆片大者，以苋菜封裹之，置于土坑内，上以土盖之，一宿尽变成鳖儿也。

（四）又，五月五日采苋菜和马齿苋为末，等分，调与妊娠，服之易产。

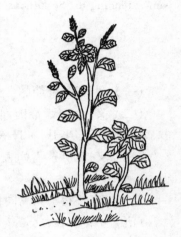

【注释】

[1] 鳖症：病症名，多由脾胃虚弱、饮食不节所致，主要症状为：症块固定不移，少腹切痛，甚则痛连腰背、面目黑黄。

## 173. Xian（Xiancai）[苋（苋菜），amaranth, Amaranthi Caulis et Folium]

It can tonify qi and clear heat. Its seeds, harvested after the Frost's Descent in the ninth lunar month, can improve vision.

Its leaves may stir qi, cause vexation and oppression, make the spleen and stomach contract coldness and impair the stomach and intestines.

It should not be taken with the turtle flesh, because it may cause turtle fixed abdominal mass[1]. Putting the turtle shell in the size of a bean wrapped and sealed by it into a pit and covering it with soil for one night can transform the small turtle shell into young turtle.

Harvest it and Machixian [马齿苋, purslane, Portulacae Herba] on the fifth day of the fifth lunar month and make them into powder respectively. Taking the equal amount of these powders together can help the pregnant women deliver smoothly.

【Note】

[1] turtle fixed abdominal mass: A disease. It is mainly caused by the spleen-stomach deficiency and dietary irregularities and characterized by the motionlessness of

concretion lumps. The patients with the disease at the moderate level can sense the abdominal pain while the patients with the disease at the severe level may have the pain extending to the lumbus and back and the face will turn black and yellow.

# 174. 胡 荽[1] 平

（一）利五藏，补筋脉。主消谷能食。若食多，则令人多忘。

（二）又，食着诸毒肉，吐、下血不止，顿瘕黄者：取净胡荽子一升，煮使腹破，取汁停冷，服半升，一日一夜二服即止。

（三）又，狐臭䘌齿病人不可食，疾更加。久冷人食之，脚弱。患气，弥不得食。

（四）又，不得与斜蒿同食。食之令人汗臭，难瘥。

（五）不得久食，此是薰菜，损人精神。

（六）秋冬捣子，醋煮熨肠头出，甚效。

（七）可和生菜食，治肠风。热饼裹食甚良。

（八）利五藏不足，不可多食，损神。

（九）味辛温，微毒。消谷，治五藏，补不足；利大小肠，通小腹气，拔四肢热，止头痛，疗沙疹、豌豆疮[2]不出，作酒喷之立出。通心窍，久食令人多忘。发腋臭、脚气。

（十）根：发痼疾。

（十一）子：主小儿秃疮，油煎敷之。亦主蛊、五痔及食肉中毒下血：煮，冷取汁服。并州[3]人呼为"香荽"。入药炒用。

**【注释】**

［1］胡荽：又名"香菜"，为伞形科植物鞠荽的全草，一、二年生草本植物，是人们熟悉的提味蔬菜，汤、饮中的佐料。

［2］豌豆疮：即天花，一种急性传染病。症状为先发高热，全身起红色丘疹，继而变成疱疹，最后成脓疱。十天左右结痂，痂脱后留有疤痕，俗称"麻子"。本病现已消灭。

［3］并州：为古九州之一，山西省会太原市旧称。

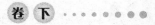
## 174. Husui[1] [胡荽, coriander herb with root, Herba Coriandri Sativicum Radice] *mild*

It can replenish the five zang-organs, supplement the sinews and vessels, aid the digestion of the five grains and increase appetite. Taking it too much may cause amnesia.

Decoct 1 Sheng of its clean seeds with water until the shells crack and pour it out to cool down. Those who have quickly-withered yellow complexion due to the incessant ejection and precipitation of blood caused by intake of all kinds of toxic meats can take half a Sheng of the decoction every time. Taking the same amount of the decoction twice a day can staunch the bleeding.

Those who have foxy smell and tooth decay should not take it, because it can make their symptoms worse. Those who contract deficiency cold for a long time should not take it, because it may weaken their feet and legs. Those who have qi disease should not take it either.

It can not be taken with Xiehao [斜蒿, seseli, Seseli Herba], because it may cause smelly sweat which is hard to cure.

Due to its pungent taste, it should not be taken often because it may impair the spirit.

In autumn and winter, pound the seeds of Husui [胡荽, coriander herb with root, Herba Coriandri Sativicum Radice], boil them with vinegar and wrap them with gauze. Then applying them externally and warmly to the tip of the large intestine which prolapses out of the anus can treat the prolapse of the rectum effectively.

Taking it with fresh vegetables can treat intestinal wind. Taking it wrapped by hot cakes is better.

It can supplement and boost the insufficiency of the five zang-organs. However, it should not be taken too much because it may impair the spirit.

Husui [胡荽, coriander herb with root, Herba Coriandri Sativicum Radice], warm (there is another saying that it is slightly cold in property) and slightly toxic in property, can transform five grains, regulate the five zang-organs, tonify and replenish insufficiency, promote the large and small intestines, dredge the stagnant qi in the smaller abdomen, disperse evil heat in the limbs and relieve headache. Those suffering from rubella and smallpox[2] that can not exude the pustule can put Husui〔胡荽, coriander herb with root, Herba Coriandri Sativicum Radice〕into liquor and spray them onto the affected area. The problem will be solved instantly. It can free the orifice of heart, but taking it often may cause amnesia. It can cause armpit odor and beriberi.

Its root may cause obstinate diseases.

The seeds: They can treat bald scalp sores on children's heads by applying the oil-fried ones externally. It can also treat the precipitation of blood caused by the parasitic toxin, the five hemorrhoids and the toxin due to intake of meat by taking its cool decoction. It is also called as "Xiangsui" in Bingzhou[3]. It should be fried if used as a drug.

**【Notes】**

〔1〕Husui: It is also called "Xiangcai", an annual or biennial herb, the whole grass of Jusui〔鞠荽, coriander, Coriandrum Sativum〕which is a species of Genus Umbelliferae. It is a common vegetable, usually used as a seasoning in soup and drink.

〔2〕smallpox: A kind of acute epidemic disease, which is characterized by first high fever and red rashes all over the whole body, and then blebs and finally exusion of pustules. The affected area will form crusts about ten days later. After decrustation, the affected area will have scars which are also called "Pockmark". However, this disease has already been eliminated nowadays.

〔3〕Bingzhou: One of the nine states in ancient times. It is the old name for "Taiyuan", the capital of Shanxi Province.

# 175. 邪 蒿[1]

味辛,温,平,无毒。似青蒿细软。主胸膈中臭烂恶邪气。利肠胃,通血脉,续不足气。生食微动风气,作羹食良。不与胡荽同食,令人汗臭气。

**【注释】**

〔1〕邪蒿:多年生草本,有利肠胃、通血脉等功效。

## 175. Xiehao[1] [邪蒿, seseli, Seseli Herba]

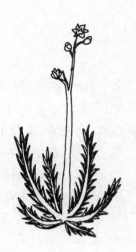

It is pungent in taste and warm, mild and non-toxic in property. Its stems are similar to those of Qinghao [青蒿, sweet wormwood, Artemisiae Annuae Herba], but thinner and softer than them. It can treat the rotten malign qi and the evil qi in the chest and diaphragm, regulate the stomach and intestines, free the blood vessels, continue and supplement the insufficient qi dynamic. Taking it raw may slightly cause the wind qi while taking it as soup is good. It should not be taken with Husui [胡荽, coriander herb with root, Herba Coriandri Sativicum Radice] because this kind of mixture can cause the stinky sweat.

【Note】

[1] Xiehao: A perennial herb. It has the effects of benefiting the stomach and intestines and freeing the blood vessels.

## 176. 同　蒿[1] 平

主安心气,养脾胃,消水饮。又,动风气,熏人心,令人气满,不可多食。

【注释】

[1] 同蒿:菊科一年生或二年生草本植物,茎叶嫩时可食,亦可入药。

## 176. Tonghao[1] [同蒿, garland chry, Chrysanthemum Coronarium] *mild*

It can quiet the heart qi, nourish the spleen and stomach and eliminate water-rheum. It can also cause the wind qi. Its flavor irritates the heart and causes the qi oppression. So it should not be taken too much.

【Note】

[1] Tonghao: An annual herbaceous plant or a biennial herbaceous plant of the Asteraceae family. Its young stems and leaves are edible and can be used as drugs.

# 177. 罗 勒

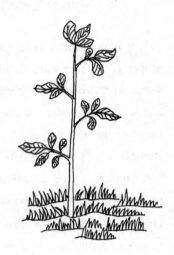

（一）味辛，温，微毒。调中消食，去恶气，消水气，宜生食。又，疗齿根烂疮，为灰用甚良。不可过多食，壅关节，涩荣卫，令血脉不行。又，动风发脚气。患啘，取汁服半合，定。冬月用干者煮之。

（二）子：主目翳及物入目，三五颗致目中，少顷当湿胀，与物俱出。又，疗风赤眵泪。

（三）根：主小儿黄烂疮，烧灰敷之佳。北人呼为"兰香"，为石勒[1]讳也。

【注释】

［1］石勒（274—333 年）：羯族，是中国晋朝时期十六国中后赵的建立者。

## 177. Luole［罗勒，basil，Basilici Herba］

It is pungent in taste and warm and slightly toxic in property. It can regulate the spleen and stomach, aid digestion, expel the malign qi and disperse the water qi. It is proper to take it raw. It can treat the ulcerated sores in the root of teeth by applying its burnt ash externally. It should not be taken too much, because it may congest the joints, astringe Rongwei and block the blood vessels. It can also cause wind qi and weak foot. Taking half a Ge of its juice can stop the dry retching, the same is true of taking the decoction of dry Luole［罗勒，basil，Basilici Herba］ in winter.

Its seeds can treat the eye screen and foreign bodies in the eyes. Put three to five seeds into the eyes for a while and then the swelling and wet seeds can stick the foreign bodies out of the eyes with them. They can still treat the red eyes with tears and too much eye discharge caused by the wind-heat invasion.

Burning its roots into ash and applying it externally can treat the yellow and ulcerated sores on children's bodies, which is very effective. Northerners also refer to it as "Lanxiang" to avoid the taboo of the name of Shile[1].

**【Notes】**

[1] Shile (274 – 333)：Jie nationality, the founder of the later Zhao, a state of the Sixteen Kingdoms during the Jin Dynasty in China.

## 178. 石胡荽[1] 寒

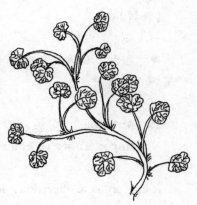

无毒。通鼻气,利九窍,吐风痰,不任食。亦去翳,熟挼内鼻中,翳自落。俗名"鹅不食草"。

**【注释】**

[1] 石胡荽:菊科一年生草本植物,喜生于潮湿的环境,是常见杂草。

**178. Shihusui[1]** [石胡荽, **myriogyne minuta less, Centipeda Minima**] *cold*

It is non-toxic in property. It can promote the nasal function, dredge the nine orifices and help expectorate the wind phlegm. But it cannot be taken as food. It can eliminate the eye nebula membrane. Rub it repeatedly and put it into the nasal cavity, and then the eye nebula membrane can shed on its own. Its trivial name is Ebushi Cao [鹅不食草, centipede, Centipedae Herba].

**【Note】**

[1] Shihusui：An annual herbaceous plant of the Asteraceae family. It favors the damp growing environment and is the common weed.

## 179. 蔓菁[1] 温

(一)消食,下气,治黄疸,利小便,根主消渴,治热毒风肿。食,令人气胀满。

(二)其子:九蒸九暴,捣为粉,服之长生。压油,涂头,能变蒜发。

(三)又,研子入面脂,极去皱。

(四)又,捣子,水和服,治热黄、结实不通,少顷当泻一切恶物,沙石草发并出。又利小便。

（五）又，女子妒乳肿，取其根生捣后，和盐醋浆水煮，取汁洗之，五、六度瘥。又捣和鸡子白封之，亦妙。

【注释】

[1] 蔓菁：又名"大头菜"，能形成肉质根的二年生草本植物。肥大肉质根可食用，有开胃下气、利湿解毒等功效。

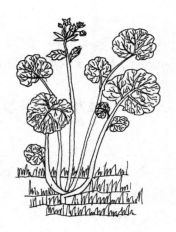

## 179. Manjing[1] [蔓菁, turnip, Brassicae Rapae Tuber et Folium] *warm*

It can promote digestion, lower qi, treat jaundice and disinhibit urine. Its roots can treat the consumptive thirst, heat toxin and rubella. Taking them can cause the qi stagnation, distention and fullness.

Seeds: Steam and expose them to the sun in turn for nine times, and then pound them into powder. Taking them can prolong life. It can treat the premature graying by applying their extracted oil to the head externally.

It can also eliminate the wrinkles on the face effectively by using the grease with its powder in it.

It can treat the excess heat, jaundice and constipation by taking the pounded one with water. A little while after that, all the nasty and muddy waste, along with the sands, stones, weeds and hair are excreted out. It can also disinhibit urine.

Boil the pounded roots of Manjing [蔓菁, turnip, Brassicae Rapae Tuber et Folium] with salt, vinegar and sour millet water. Washing the affected area with the decoction five or six times can cure women's swelling of breasts. Applying the pounded roots with egg white still has great effects.

【Note】

[1] Manjing: It is also known as Datoucai [大头菜, kohlrabi, Brassicae Caulorapae Cormus], a biennial herb with fleshy roots. Its fleshy roots are edible and have the effects of increasing the appetite, lowering qi, disinhibiting dampness and resolving toxin.

# 180. 冬 瓜<sup>[1]</sup> 寒

（一）右主治小腹水鼓胀<sup>[2]</sup>。

（二）又，利小便，止消渴。

（三）又，其子：主益气耐老，除心胸气满，消痰止烦。

（四）又，冬瓜子七升，（以）绢袋盛（之），投三沸汤中，须臾（出），曝干，又内汤中，如此三度乃止。曝干。与清苦酒浸之一宿，曝干为末，服之方寸匕，日二服，令人肥悦。

（五）又，明目，延年不老。

（六）案经：压丹石，去头面热风。

（七）又，热发者服之良。患冷人匆食之，令人益瘦。

（八）取冬瓜一颗，和桐叶与猪食之。一冬更不食诸物，（自然不饥），其猪肥长三、四倍矣。

（九）又，煮食之，能炼五藏精细。欲得肥者，勿食之，欲瘦小轻健者，食之甚健人。

（十）又，冬瓜人三（五）升，退去皮壳，（捣）为丸。空腹及食后各服廿丸，令人面滑静如玉。可入面脂中用。

【注释】

［1］冬瓜：葫芦科一年生蔓生草本植物，味甘，性寒，有消热、利水、消肿等功效。

［2］水鼓胀：病症名，是历代中医"风、痨、鼓、膈"四大疑难症之一，本病病机主要为肝脾肾三脏俱病，气血水淤积于腹内。现代医学的肝硬化腹水、晚期血吸虫病形成的腹水等，都属该病范围。

## 180. Donggua<sup>[1]</sup> [冬瓜, wax gourd, Benincasae Fructus] *cold*

It can treat the water tympanites<sup>[2]</sup> in the smaller abdomen.

It can disinhibit urine and quench the consumptive thirst.

Its seeds can replenish qi, decelerate aging, disperse the qi staganation, fullness and oppression in the heart and chest, eliminate phlegm and stop vexation.

Bring the water to boiling three times and put a silk bag of 7 Sheng of its seeds into water for a little while, and then take it out and dry it in the sun. Repeat the procedure three times and dry it finally. Steep it in the vinegar for one night, dry it in the sun and grind it into powder. Taking 1 Fangcunbi (square-cun-spoon) of the powder every time and twice a day can make people fat and happy.

It can also improve vision and prolong life.

The following is supplemented by Zhang Ding: It can inhibit the Danshi toxin, eliminate the wind heat in the face and head.

Those who catch fever can take it, because it has good effects of treating this disease. Those who get the deficiency cold should not take it, because it can make them emaciated.

Feed a pig with one Donggua [冬瓜, wax gourd, Benincasae Fructus] as well as Tongye [桐叶, paulownia leaf, Paulowniae Folium]. The pig will not feel hungry for the whole winter even without taking any other food, and it may gain weight three times or four times as much as it used to have.

Taking the boiled one can regulate essential qi in the five zang-organs. The thin people who want to put on weight should not take it because it can lower qi. Those who want to lose weight and become slim can take it because it can make people athletic.

Take 3 or 5 Sheng of its seeds. Unhusk the shells, pound them and make them into pills. Taking twenty pills before meals and after meals respectively can make the facial skin as smooth and delicate as the jade. The pills can also be put into the grease to use.

【Notes】

[1] Donggua: A Cucurbitaceous annual bine plant, sweet in taste and cold in property, has the effects of eliminating heat, disinhibiting water and dispersing swelling.

[2] water tympanites: A disease. It is one of the four difficult and complicated diseases in the Traditional Chinese Medicine which are "wind, tuberculosis, tympanites and diaphragm". The pathogenesis of this disease is that the liver, the spleen and the kidney are all diseased, thus qi, water and blood are stagnated in the abdomen. The liver cirrhosis ascites and the ascites caused by schistosomiasis in modern medicine belong to this category.

# 181. 濮 瓜[1]

孟诜说:肺热消渴,取濮瓜去皮,每食后嚼吃三二两,五七度良。

**【注释】**

[1] 濮瓜:冬瓜的别名,可以拿来煮汤,又可以炒食。有减肥、润肺等功效。

## 181. Pugua[1][濮瓜, wax gourd, Benincasae Fructus]

Meng Shen said, "It can treat the lung heat and the consumptive thirst by taking 2 or 3 Liang of the peeled one after each meal. It will have great effects if taken in this way five or seven times in succession.

**【Note】**

[1] Pugua: It is also known as Donggua[冬瓜, white gourd, Benincasa hispida] and can be used to make soup or fry. It has the effects of losing weight and moistening the lung.

# 182. 甜 瓜[1] 寒

(一)右止渴,(益气),除烦热。多食令人阴下痒湿、生疮。

(二)又,发瘅黄,动宿冷病,患症瘕人不可食瓜。(若食之饱胀,入水自消。)

(三)其瓜蒂:主治身面四肢浮肿,杀蛊,去鼻中瘜肉,阴瘅黄及急黄[2]。

(四)又,生瓜叶:捣取汁,治人头不生毛发者,涂之即生。

(五)案经:多食令人羸惙虚弱,脚手少力。其子热,补中焦,宜人。其肉止渴,利小便,通三焦间拥塞气。

(六)又方,瓜蒂七枚,丁香七枚,(小豆七粒),捣为末,吹(黑豆许于)鼻中,少时治癃气,黄汁即出,瘥。

(七)又,补中打损折,碾末酒服去瘀血,治小儿疳。《龙鱼河图》云:瓜有两鼻者杀人;沉水者杀人;食多饱胀,可食盐,化成水。

(八)寒,有毒。止渴,除烦热,多食令人阴下湿痒、生疮。动宿冷病,发虚热,破腹。又,令人惙惙弱,脚手无力。少食即止渴,利小便,通三焦间拥塞气。

兼主口鼻疮。

（九）叶：治人无发，捣汁涂之即生。

【注释】

［1］甜瓜：葫芦科黄瓜属一年生蔓生草本植物，味甘，性寒，有清暑热、解烦渴、利小便等功效。

［2］阴㿌黄及急黄：阴㿌黄，病症名，指无热恶寒，小便自利，全身呈黄色不鲜明的黄疸。急黄，亦称"瘟黄"，属黄疸范畴，是一种非常险恶的急性传染病，症见高热烦渴、小便赤黄、突然面目发黄。

## 182. Tiangua[1]［甜瓜，melon，Melonis Fructus］ *cold*

It can quench thirst, replenish qi and disperse the heat vexation. Taking it too much may cause the itch, dampness and sores in the genital region.

It can also cause the jaundice and old deficiency cold. The people with the abdominal mass should not take it. If taking it too much to bloat, people can bathe in the water to eliminate the abdominal swelling.

Its stalk can treat the puffy swelling in the face and limbs, kill the mysterious toxin, eliminate the nasal polyp and treat the yin jaundice and the acute jaundice[2].

It can treat baldness and make the hair grow by applying the pounded juice of its raw leaves.

The following is supplemented by Zhang Ding：Taking it too much can make people emaciated and fatigue and weaken the limbs. Its seeds, hot in property, can replenish and tonify the middle energizer and benefit people. Its flesh can quench thirst, disinhibit urine and free the stagnant qi in the triple energizer.

Pound the mixture of seven stalks of it, seven Dingxiang ［丁香, clove, Caryophylli Flos］ and seven Xiaodou ［小豆, black gram, Phaseoli Mungo Semen］ into powder. Blowing the powder of the amount in the size of a Heidou ［黑豆, black soybean, Sojae Semen Atrum］ into the nose a little while can expel the congested qi in the nose and make the yellow mucus flow out.

It can tonify the middle and treat knocks, falls and fractures. It can eliminate the static blood and treat the infantile malnutrition by taking its ground powder with liquor. *Long Yu He Tu*［《龙鱼河图》, *River Chart from Dragon and Fish*］states that those with two stalks have deadly toxin and those that can sink to the bottom of water have deadly toxin too. If taking it too much to bloat, people can take some salt to dissolve it into water.

It is toxic and cold in property. It can quench thirst and disperse the heat vexation. Taking it too much may cause the itch, dampness and sores in the genital region. It can cause the old deficiency cold, deficiency heat and diarrhea. It can also cause emaciation and fatigue and weaken the limbs. It can quench thirst, disinhibit urine, free the stagnant qi in the triple energizer and treat the oral and nasal sores if taken a little.

It can treat baldness and make the hair grow by applying the pounded juice of its leaves.

**【Note】**

［1］Tiangua：A Cucurbitaceous annual bine plant, which is a species of Genus Cucumis, sweet in taste and cold in property, has the effects of eliminating the summer heat, relieving the vexation thirst and disinhibiting urine.

［2］the yin jaundice and the acute jaundice：yin jaundice, a disease referring to the jaundice with no-fever cold aversion, uninhibited urination and unbright yellow color. Acute jaundice, a dangerous infectious disease with the symptoms of high fever, vexation and thirst, deep-colored urine and sudden yellow appearance.

## 183. 胡 瓜[1] 寒

（一）不可多食,动风及寒热。又发疳疟[2],兼积瘀血。

（二）案:多食令人虚热上气,生百病,消人阴,发疮（疥）,及发痃气,及脚气,损血脉。天行后不可食。

（三）小儿食,发痢,滑中,生疳虫。

（四）又,不可和酪食之,必再发。

（五）又,捣根敷胡刺毒肿,甚良。

（六）叶:味苦,平,小毒。主小儿闪癖[3]:一岁服一叶,已上斟酌与之。生授绞汁服,得吐、下。

（七）根:捣敷胡刺毒肿。

（八）其实：味甘,寒,有毒。不可多食,动寒热,多疟病,积瘀热,发痓气,令人虚热上逆,少气,发百病及疮疥,损阴血脉气,发脚气。天行后不可食。小儿切忌,滑中,生疳虫。不与醋同食。北人亦呼为黄瓜,为石勒讳,因而不改。

**【注释】**

[1] 胡瓜：黄瓜,葫芦科一年生蔓生草本植物,有清热、解渴、利水、消肿等功效。

[2] 痁疟：病名,疟疾的一种。

[3] 小儿闪癖：病名,多指小孩头发竖立、面色发黄、瘦弱。

## 183. Hugua[1] [胡瓜, cucumber, Cucumeris Sativi Fructus] *cold*

It cannot be taken too much, because it may cause the wind qi, deficiency cold, heat disease and heat malaria[2] and accumulate the static blood.

The following is supplemented by Zhang Ding: It may cause the deficiency heat, the qi ascent, all kinds of diseases, impair the sexual function, cause sores, scabs, strings and aggregations, weak foot and damage the blood vessels if taken too much. Those who contract the epidemic should not take it, because it may cause the epidemic again.

Children should not take it, because it may cause dysentery, the efflux diarrhea of the middle energizer and the infantile malnutrition due to worms.

It should not be taken with cheese, because this mixture may cause the old disease.

It can effectively treat the toxic swellings caused by the thorns whose surface is covered with the fox's urine by applying its pounded roots externally to the wounds.

Its leaves, bitter in taste and mild and slightly toxic in property, can treat children's Shanpi[3]. The children aged one year old with Shanpi can take one leaf; those older than one year old can take the amount due to the specific situation. Children may take the juice rubbed and ground from its fresh leaves. After that, if they can vomit, the disease will be eliminated totally.

Root: It can treat the toxic swellings caused by the thorns whose surface is covered with the fox's urine by applying its pounded roots externally to the wounds.

Its fruit is sweet in taste and cold and toxic in property. It should not be taken too much because it can cause the deficiency cold, heat disease and malaria, accumulate the static heat, cause the infixation qi, vacuity heat, qi ascending counterflow, shortness of breath, all kinds of diseases, sores and scabs, impair the sexual function, blood vessels and qi movement and cause weak foot. Those who contract epidemic should not take it. Children should not take it, because it may cause the efflux diarrhea of the middle energizer and infantile malnutrition due to worms. It should not be taken with vinegar. Northerners call it as "Huanggua" to avoid the taboo of the title of "Shile". This name is used to present and never changes back.

**【Notes】**

[1] Hugua：It is also known as Cucumber, Cucurbitaceous annual bine plant, which has the effects of eliminating heat, relieving thirst, disinhibiting water and dispersing swelling.

[2] heat malaria：A disease. It is one kind of malarias.

[3] children's Shanpi：A disease. It is characterized by the symptoms that the children have the erect hair, yellow face and emaciated body.

# 184. 越　瓜[1] 寒

（一）右主治利阴阳，益肠胃，止烦渴，不可久食，发痢。

（二）案：此物动风。虽止渴，能发诸疮。令人虚，脚弱，虚不能行（立）。小儿夏月不可与食，成痢，发虫。令人腰脚冷，脐下痛。

（三）患时疾后不可食。

（四）不得和牛乳及酪食之。

（五）又，不可空腹和醋食之，令人心痛。

**【注释】**

[1] 越瓜：甜瓜的变种，果皮极薄，成熟之后具有香气，但缺乏甜味，性喜高温多湿，有利肠胃、止烦渴等功效。

## 184. Yuegua[1] [越瓜, Oriental pickling melon, Cucumeris Conomonis Fructus] *cold*

It can harmonize yin and yang, tonify and replenish the stomach and intestines and quench vexation and thirst. Taking it too often may cause dysentery.

The following is supplemented by Zhang Ding: It can cause the wind qi. Though quenching thirst, it may cause all kinds of sores, weaken the body and feet and cause the inability to walk and stand. Children should not take it in summer, because they may contract dysentery and have worms in the abdomen. It can make the waist and legs cold and cause pains under the umbilical region.

People should not take it after contracting the seasonal epidemic.

It should not be taken with milk and cheese.

It should not be taken with vinegar on an empty stomach, because it may cause the heart pain.

【Note】

[1] Yuegua: The variant of Tiangua [甜瓜, melon, Melonis Fructus]. Its skin is very thin. The ripe Yuegua [越瓜, Oriental pickling melon, Cucumeris Conomonis Fructus] has a flavor of fragrance but lacks sweetness. It likes the heat and damp environment and has the effects of disinhibiting the stomach and intestines and quenching the dispersion-thirst.

## 185. 芥[1]

（一）主咳逆下气，明目，去头面风。大叶者良。煮食之亦动气，犹胜诸菜。生食发丹石，不可多食。

（二）其子：微熬研之，作酱香美，有辛气，能通利五藏。

（三）其叶不可多食。又，细叶有毛者杀人。

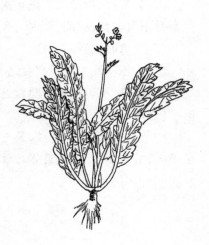

【注释】

[1] 芥:一年或二年生草本植物,种子黄色,味辛辣,磨成粉末,称为"芥末",可作调味品。

## 185. Jie[1][芥, mustard leaf, Sinapis Folium]

It can mainly treat cough and counterflow, lower qi and disperse the wind evil in the head and face. Those with large leaves are good. It may stir qi if taken boiled, but it is still better than other vegetables. It should not be taken too much and its raw one may cause the Danshi medicinal toxicity.

Boil its seeds slightly, grind them and make them into sauce. The sauce tastes delicious and has the pungent flavor, which can free and nourish the five zang-organs.

Its leaves should not be taken too much and those with small leaves and hair can kill people due to their toxin.

【Note】

[1] Jie: An annual or biennial herb. Its seeds are yellow and have the pungent flavor. Its ground powder is called mustard which is used as seasoning.

## 186. 萝卜[1](莱菔) 冷

(一) 利五藏,轻身益气。

(二) 根:消食下气。甚利关节,除五藏中风,练五藏中恶气。服之令人白净肌细。

【注释】

[1] 萝卜:十字花科一年或二年生草本植物,具有很强的行气功能,以及止咳化痰、润燥生津等功效。

## 186. Luobo[1](Laifu)［萝卜(莱菔), radish, Raphani Radix］*cold*

It can regulate and nourish the five zang-organs, relax the body and replenish qi.

Its roots can promote digestion, lower qi, disinhibit the joints, expel the wind evil in the five zang-organs and disperse the malign qi in the five zang-organs. Taking it often can make the complexion delicate and fair.

【Note】

[1] Luobo: An annual or biennial herb which belongs to the Cruciferae. It has great effects of moving qi, suppressing cough, resolving phlegm, moistening dryness and engendering liquid.

# 187. 菘　菜[1] 温

（一）治消渴。又发诸风冷。（腹中冷病者不服。）

有热者服之，亦不发病，即明其（菜）性冷。《本草》云"温"，未解。

（二）又，消食，亦少下气。

（三）九英菘，出河西，叶极大，根亦粗长。和羊肉甚美。常食之，都不见发病。其冬月作菹，煮作羹食之，能消宿食，下气治嗽。诸家商略，性冷，非温。恐误也。

（四）又，北无菘菜，南无芜菁。其蔓菁子，细；菜子，粗也。

【注释】

[1] 菘菜：大白菜，品质鲜嫩，营养丰富，既可鲜食，又能加工腌渍，为中国北方冬春的主要蔬菜。

## 187. Songcai[1]［菘菜，pakchoi，Brassicae Chinensis Herba］*warm*

It can treat the consumptive thirst and cause all kinds of diseases of wind coldness. Those who have the deficiency cold in the abdomen should not take it while those who have heat in the body can take it without contracting diseases, which is a good case to illustrate its cold property. Its warm property is recorded in *Shen Nong Ben Cao Jing*［《神农本草经》，*Agriculture God's Canon of Materia Medica*］which is hard to understand.

It can promote digestion and lower qi slightly.

Jiuyingsong［九英菘，turnip，Brassicae Rapae Tuber et Folium］，growing in Hexi，has large leaves and thick and long roots. It tastes very good when boiling with mutton. Taking it with mutton often will not cause any disease. Taking the soup of the pickled Jiuyingsong〔九英菘, turnip, Brassicae Rapae Tuber et Folium〕made in winter can digest the accumulated food in the stomach, lower qi and treat cough. Many doctors agree that its property is cold rather than warm. Those who think it warm may make a mistake.

There is no Songcai〔菘菜, pakchoi, Brassicae Chinensis Herba〕in the north while there is no Manjing〔蔓菁, turnip, Brassicae Rapae Tuber et Folium〕in the south. The latter's seeds are small and thin whereas the former's seeds are larger.

【Notes】

〔1〕Songcai：It is also known as Dabaicai〔大白菜, celery cabbage, Brassicae Pekinensis Folium〕. It is fresh, tender and rich in nutrition. It can be taken fresh and pickled, which is the major vegetable in winter and spring for the people living in the north of China.

## 188. 荏 子[1]

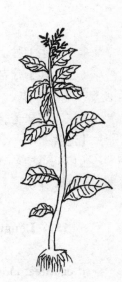

（一）主咳逆下气。

（二）其叶性温。用时捣之。治男子阴肿,生捣和醋封之。女人绵裹内,三四易。

（三）谨按:子:压作油用,亦少破气,多食发心闷。温。补中益气,通血脉,填精髓。可蒸令熟,烈日干之,当口开。春取米食之,亦可休粮。生食,止渴、润肺。

【注释】

〔1〕荏子:又名"白苏",一年生草本植物,种子可榨油,也可入药,有散寒解表、理气宽中等功效。

## 188. Renzi[1]〔荏子, white perilla, Perillae Albae〕

It can treat cough and counterflow and lower qi.

Its leaves are warm in property. Its leaves can treat the male genital swelling by applying the pounded fresh one with vinegar to the affected area and sealing it with vinegar. The same is true of the female genital swelling by putting the pounded fresh one with vinegar wrapped with silk floss into women's vagina and changing the dressings three or four times.

The following is supplemented by Zhang Ding：Taking its extracted oil may break qi a little. Taking it too much may cause the distention and oppression in the heart. It is warm in property. It can tonify the middle, replenish qi, disinhibit the blood vessels, supplement essence and replenish marrow. It can be steamed and dried under the scorching sun to crack its external shells and pounded out the kernels. The kernels can be taken and used in the period of inedia. Taking it raw can quench the consumptive thirst and moisten the lung.

【Note】

［1］Renzi：It is also known as Baisu［白苏, white perilla, Perillae Albae］, an annual herb. Its seeds can be used to extract oil and can be used as drugs. It has the effects of dissipating cold, relieving exterior, regulating qi and smoothing the center.

# 189. 龙 葵[1]

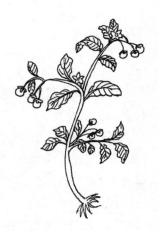

（一）主丁肿。患火丹疮,和土杵敷之尤良。

（二）其子疗甚妙。其赤珠者名龙珠,久服变发,长黑。令人不老。

（三）其味苦,皆揉去汁食之。

【注释】

［1］龙葵:一年生草本植物,全株入药,可化瘀消肿、清热解毒。

## 189. Longkui[1]［龙葵, black nightshade, Solani Nigri Herba］

It can treat clove sores. It can treat erysipelas with great effects by applying the pestle-pounded mixture of it and soil.

Its seeds also have great efficacy. Its red fruit is called as "dragon ball", which can make the hair longer and blacker and prolong life by the long-term taking of it.

Since it tastes bitter, it is often taken after ridding the juice of it via rubbing

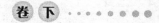

and kneading.

【Note】

　[1] Longkui：An annual herb. The whole plant can be used as drug and it can resolve stasis，disperse swelling，clear heat and resolve toxin.

# 190. 苜　蓿[1]

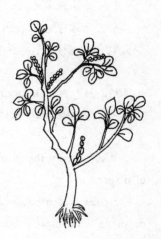

　（一）患疸黄人，取根生捣，绞汁服之良。

　（二）又，利五藏，轻身；洗去脾胃间邪气，诸恶热毒。少食好，多食当冷气入筋中，即瘦人。亦能轻身健人，更无诸益。

　（三）彼处人采根作土黄耆也。又，安中，利五藏，煮和酱食之。作羹亦得。

【注释】

　[1] 苜蓿：苜蓿属植物的通称。其种类繁多，多是野生的草本植物。其营养价值高，具有清脾胃、利大小肠、下膀胱结石等功效。

## 190. Muxu[1]［苜蓿，alfalfa，Medicaginis Herba］

It can treat jaundice with great effects by taking the juice pounded from its fresh roots.

It can replenish the five zang-organs，relax the body，eliminate evil qi in the spleen and stomach and treat all kinds of malign evil and heat toxin. It is better to take it a little，otherwise it may cause the invasion of cold qi into the muscles and tendons and gradual emaciation. It can also relax the body and make people healthy. Apart from these，there are no other benefits.

Its roots are used as Tuhuangqi［土黄芪，moghania，Moghaniae Radix］in its growing regions. It can also quiet the middle and replenish the five zang-organs. It can be taken boiled with sauce and made as soup.

【Note】

　[1] Muxu：The general term for the Genus Medicago. It has many species，

most of which are wild herbs. It is rich in nutrition and has effects of clearing the spleen and stomach, disinhibiting the large and small intestines and expelling the urethral calculi.

# 191. 荠

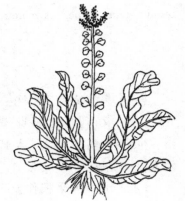

（一）补五藏不足。叶：动气。

（二）荠子：入治眼方中用。不与面同食。令人背闷。服丹石人不可食。

### 191. Ji〔荠, shepherd's purse, Capsellae Bursa-Pastoris Herba〕

It can tonify the insufficiency of the five zang-organs. Its leaves can cause the qi disease.

Its seeds can be used in the therapy of treating the eye disease. It should not be taken with flour, because it may cause the distention and oppression in the back. It should not be taken either by those who take Danshi.

# 192. 蕨[1] 寒

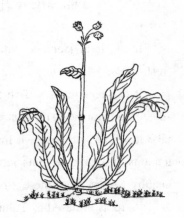

（一）补五藏不足。气壅经络筋骨间，毒气。令人脚弱不能行。消阳事，缩玉茎。多食令人发落，鼻塞，目暗。小儿不可食之，立行不得也。

（二）又，冷气人食之，多腹胀。

【注释】

〔1〕蕨：多年生草本植物，根茎长，嫩叶可食，根茎可制淀粉，全株可入药。

### 192. Jue[1]〔蕨, bracken, Pteridii Aquilini Folium〕 *cold*

It can tonify the insufficiency of the five zang-organs, treat the qi stagnation

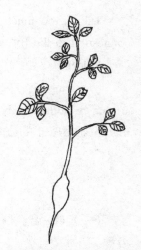

in the meridians, sinews and bones and disperse the toxic qi. It may make the feet
and legs too weak to walk, weaken men's sexual function and wither penis.
Taking it often may cause the hair loss, nasal congestion and dim vision. Children
should not take it because it may make children not able to stand and walk.

People with the cold qi should not take it because it may cause the abdominal
distention.

【Note】

[1] Jue: A perennial herb with long roots and stems. Its fresh leaves are edible.
Its roots and stems can be made into starch. The whole plant can be used as drug.

# 193. 翘摇[1]（小巢菜）

（一）疗五种黄病：生捣汁,服一升,日二,差。

（二）甚益人,和五藏,明耳目,去热风,令人轻健。
长食不厌,煮熟吃,佳。若生吃,令人吐水。

【注释】

[1] 翘摇:豆种植物硬毛果野豌豆的全草,具有解
表利湿、活血止血等功效。

## 193. Qiaoyao[1]（Xiaochaocai）［翘摇（小巢菜）, herb of tiny vetch, Viciahirsuta］

It can cure five kinds of jaundice by taking 1 Sheng of its pounded juice every
time and twice a day.

It can benefit the body a lot, harmonize the five zang-organs, improve vision
and hearing, disperse the wind heat, relax the body and make it strong. The long-
term taking of it does not bore people. Taking it boiled is good. Taking it raw may
cause the water vomiting.

【Note】

[1] Qiaoyao: The whole grass of the vetch which is a kind of hard and hairy
fruit and belongs to the soybean plant. It has the effects of relieving exterior and
eliminating dampness, and activating blood and stopping bleeding.

## 194. 蓼子(蓼实)

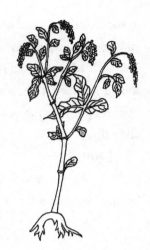

多食令人吐水。亦通五藏拥气,损阳气[1]。

【注释】

[1] 阳气:充盈于周身之气,具有温养组织脏器、维持生理功能、固卫体表等作用。

## 194. Liaozi (Liaoshi) 〔蓼子(蓼实), red knees fruit, Fructus Polygoni Hydropiperis〕

Taking too much of it may cause the water vomiting. It can remove qi congestion in the five zang-organs. It can also impair yang qi[1].

【Note】

[1] yang qi: The term in Traditional Chinese Medicine refers to the qi flowing around in human body which can warm and tonify the tissues and organs, maintain the physiological functions and consolidate the exterior.

## 195. 葱[1] 温

(一)叶:温。白:平。主伤寒壮热、出汗;中风,面目浮肿,骨节头疼,损发鬓。

(二)葱白及须:平。通气,主伤寒头痛。

(三)又,治疮中有风水,肿疼、秘涩:取青叶同干姜、黄蘗相和,煮作汤,浸洗之,立愈。

(四)冬葱最善,宜冬月食,不宜多。只可和五味用之。虚人患气者,多食发气,上冲人,五藏闭绝,虚人胃。开骨节,出汗,故温尔。

(五)少食则得,可作汤饮。不得多食,恐拔气上冲人,五藏闷绝。切不可与蜜相和,食之促人气,杀人。

(六)又,止血衄[2],利小便。

【注释】

[1] 葱:百合科葱属多年生草本植物,喜冷凉,不耐炎热,有解热祛痰、防癌

抗癌等功效。

[2] 血衄:病症名,常指非外伤性所致的头部诸窍及肌表出血,此处为鼻出血。

## 195. Cong[1] [葱, scallion, Allii Fistulosi Herba] *warm*

Its leaves are warm in property. Its white is mild in property. It can treat the cold damage, vigorous heat, sweat, wind stroke, puffy swelling of the face and eyes, joints' pains and headache. It may impair the hair.

Its white and root, mild in property, can free the qi dynamic and treat the cold damage and headache.

It can treat the wind water, the swelling and pain of sores and the situation that the infected wounds do not evacuate pus by decocting its green leaves with dried ginger and Huangnie [黄蘗, phellodendron, Phellodendri Cortex], bathing and watering the infected area with this decoction.

Those harvested in winter are the best and suitable for being taken in winter. However, it should not be taken too much. It is suitable to be taken with all kinds of seasonings. It may cause the qi disease, the surging up of counterflow qi and blockage of the five zang-organs and weaken the stomach qi if taken too much by the people who are weak and have the qi disease. Since it can free the joints and make people sweat, so it is warm in property.

It is agreeable to be taken a little, and it can be made into soup. It should not be taken too much, because it may cause the surging up of the counterflow qi and the blockage of the five zang-organs. Do remember: It cannot be taken with honey, because this mixture may cause tachypnea or even claim life.

It can stop epistaxis[2] and free urine.

**[ Notes ]**

[1] Cong: A scallion species of Genus liliaceae, perennial herb. It likes the cold environment and cannot stand the heat. It has the effects of resolving heat, dispelling phlegm and anti-cancer.

[2] epistaxis: The name of a disease, usually it refers to the non-traumatic bleeding from orifices in the head and muscle surface. Here it refers to nasal bleeding.

# 196. 韭

（一）冷气人，可煮，长服之。

（二）热病后十日，不可食热韭，食之即发困。

（三）又，胸痹[1]，心中急痛如锥刺，不得俯仰，白汗出。或痛彻背不治或至死：可取生韭或根五斤，洗，捣汁灌少许，即吐胸中恶血。

（四）亦可作菹，空心食之，甚验。此物炸熟，以盐、醋空心吃一楪，可十顿已上。甚治胸膈咽气，利胸膈，甚验。

（五）初生孩子，可捣根汁灌之，即吐出胸中恶血，永无诸病。

（六）五月勿食韭。若值时馑之年，可与米同功。种之一亩[2]，可供十口食。

**【注释】**

[1] 胸痹：病症名。胸部闷痛，甚则胸痛彻背，喘息不得卧，轻者感觉胸闷，呼吸欠畅，重者则有胸痛，严重者心痛彻背，背痛彻心。正气亏虚、气滞、寒凝、血瘀导致心脉痹阻不畅、瘀血阻弱，引起心脏失养。

[2] 亩：市制土地面积单位，一亩等于大约 667 平方米。

## 196. Jiu［韭，Chinese leek，Allium Tuberosum Rottler］

The people suffering from cold qi can take the boiled Jiu［韭，Chinese leek，Allium Tuberosum Rottler］for a long term.

Do not eat the hot Jiu［韭，Chinese leek，Allium Tuberosum Rottler］within ten days after suffering from the heat diseases as it will cause fatigue.

Suffering from the chest impediment[1] will feel the acute pain like the piercing of an awl in the chest, unable to bend forward and backward with the vacuity sweating, or feel the pain stretching through to the back, which may cause death if not treated. To treat the pain, take 5 Jin of fresh Jiu［韭，Chinese leek，Allium Tuberosum Rottler］or its root, wash it, crush it to extract the juice and take a little juice, and then the malign blood will be ejected.

It can be made into sauerkraut. Taking it on an empty stomach is quite effective. After blanching it, add in salt and vinegar and take one saucer of it for

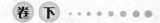

over ten times, which is very effective in treating the qi stagnation in the chest and diaphragm and disinhibiting the chest and diaphragm.

Feeding the newborn infants with the juice of its roots can help eject the malign blood in the chest and prevent suffering from the various diseases thereafter.

Do not eat it in the fifth lunar month. In case of the famine year, it can be taken to relieve hunger as the rice does. 1 Mu[2] of Jiu〔韭, Chinese leek, Allium Tuberosum Rottler〕can feed a family of ten people.

【Notes】

〔1〕chest impediment: The name of a disease pattern. Patients will feel the oppressive pain in the chest, even with the pain in the whole back and panting making it hard to lie down. The less severe patients have the thoracic oppression and short breathing; the more severe patients have chest pain stretching through to the back and back pain stretching through to the chest. The depletion of the right qi, qi stagnation, congealing cold and blood stasis causes the heart vessels obstruction, the static blood obstructing the network vessels and thus causes heart deprived of nourishment.

〔2〕Mu: A unit of land measure in ancient times. 1 Mu is about 667 square meters.

# 197. 薤[1]

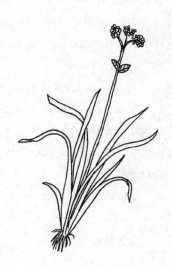

（一）轻身耐老。疗金疮、生肌肉：生捣薤白，以火封之。更以火就炙，令热气彻疮中，干则易之。

（二）疗诸疮中风水肿，生捣，热涂上，或煮之。

（三）白色者最好。虽有辛气，不荤人五藏。

（四）又，发热病，不宜多食。三月勿食生者。

（五）又，治寒热，去水气，温中，散结气：可作羹。

（六）（心腹胀满）：可作宿菹，空腹食之。

（七）又，治女人赤白带下。

（八）学道人长服之，可通神灵，甚安魂魄，益气,续筋力。

（九）骨鲠在咽不去者,食之即下。

【注释】

［1］薤(xiè):又名"藠头""薤白头""野蒜",为多年生草本百合科植物的地下鳞茎,也可食用,有通阳散结、行气导滞之效。

## 197. Xie[1]［薤, Chinese chive, Allii Macrostemonis Bulbus］

Taking it can make a man full of vigor and prevent aging. It can be used to treat the injury caused by metal and engender muscles. Smash the fresh bulb of it, warm it with fire, apply it to the sore and fire-cure it to make the heat penetrate into the sores. Change a new one when it dries.

To treat the various swollen sores caused by the wind evil, smash the fresh Xie［薤, Chinese chive, Allii Macrostemonis Bulbus］, warm it and apply it to the sores, or boil it out and apply it to the sores.

The white one has the best quality. Although it is pungent in taste, it doesn't interfere with the functions of the five zang-organs.

It can cause the heat disease, so don't eat it excessively. Don't eat the fresh one in the third lunar month.

The soup made of it can be used to treat the aversion to cold with fever, eliminate the water qi, warm the middle and disperse qi stagnation.

Eating the overnight pickled Xie［薤, Chinese chive, Allii Macrostemonis Bulbus］ on an empty stomach can treat the distention and fullness in the heart and abdomen.

It can be used to treat the red and white vaginal discharge.

The people who intend to cultivate immortality can take it for a long term, which can enable them to communicate with the gods. It can be used to greatly pacify the ethereal soul and corporeal soul, replenish qi and increase energy and strength.

To take out the bone stuck in the throat, take it and the bone will be swallowed.

【Note】

［1］Xie: Also known as Jiaotou（藠头）, Xiebaitou（薤白头）, or Yesuan

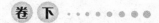

（野蒜）. It is a perennial herbaceous plant, the genus of the Liliaceae. Its bulbs can be used as drugs and are edible. It is effective in activating yang and dissipating binds, moving qi and removing the food stagnation.

## 198. 荆芥[1]（假苏） 温

（一）辟邪气,除劳,传送五藏不足气,助脾胃。多食薰人五藏神。通利血脉,发汗,动渴疾[2]。

（二）又,杵为末,醋和封风毒肿上。

（三）患丁肿,荆芥一把,水五升,煮取二升,冷,分二服。

（四）荆芥一名菥蓂。

【注释】

［1］荆芥:又名"假苏""菥蓂",是唇形科、荆芥属多年生植物,味平,性温,无毒,清香气浓。荆芥为发汗、解热药,是中华常用草药之一,能镇痰、祛风、凉血。

［2］渴疾:一种类似西病中的糖尿病的一种疾病,以多尿、多饮、烦渴、消瘦或尿有甜味为典型临床表现。

### 198. Jingjie[1]（Jiasu）［荆芥（假苏）, fineleaf schizonepeta herb, Herba Schizonepetae］ *warm*

It is used to repel the evil qi, eliminate fatigue, activate insufficient qi of the five zang-organs and fortify the spleen and stomach. Taking it excessively can interfere with the functions of the five zang-organs. It can be used to disinhibit the blood vessels and induce sweating. But it can also cause the consumptive thirst[2].

To treat the toxic swelling or the swelling caused by wind evil, grind it into powder, mix it with vinegar and apply it to the swelling.

To treat the clove sore, decoct a handful of it with 5 Sheng of water into 2 Sheng of decoction, and take it two times in equal amount after it gets cool.

It is also known as Ximi（菥蓂）.

【Notes】

［1］Jingjie: Also known as Jiasu or Ximi, a perennial plant of the Nepeta, the genus of the Lamiaceae. It is bland in taste, warm in property and non-toxic with thick delicate fragrance. As a commonly used medicinal herb, it is effective in inducing sweating, clearing heat, resolving phlegm, expelling wind and cooling blood.

[2] consumptive thirst: A disease similar to the diabetes in the Western medicine, characterized by polydipsia, polyphagia, polyuria, emaciation or sweet urine.

## 199. 莙 菜[1]

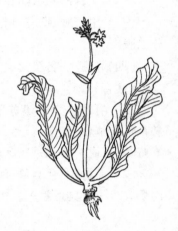

（一）又,捣汁与时疾人服,瘥。

（二）子:煮半生,捣取汁,含,治小儿热。

【注释】

[1] 莙菜:藜科,属二年生草本植物,味甘,性平,通经脉,下气,开胸膈。

### 199. Tiancai[1]［莙菜, spinach beet, Betae Ciclae Caulis et Folium］

The patients with seasonal epidemics can take juice extracted from crushing it, and then the disease will be cured.

Boil its seeds to half-done and crush them to extract juice. Holding the juice in mouth can treat the fever in children.

【Note】

[1] Tiancai: The genus of the Chenopodiaceae, a biennal herbaceous plant. Sweet in taste and mild in property, it can free the meridians, lower qi and disinhibit the chest and diaphragm.

## 200. 紫　苏[1]

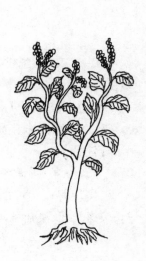

除寒热,治冷气。

【注释】

[1]紫苏:唇形科一年生草本植物。气清香,味微辛。叶能散表寒,发汗力较强,用于风寒表症,见恶寒、发热、无汗等症,常配生姜同用。

## 200. Zisu[1]［紫苏, perilla, Perillae Folium, Caulis et Calyx］

It can eliminate cold and heat, and treat cold qi.

【Note】

[1] Zisu: An annual herbaceous plant, the genus of the Lamiaceae. Slightly bitter in taste with fragrance, its leaves can dissipate exterior cold and are very effective in inducing sweating. It is used to treat the wind-cold exterior pattern with the symptoms like the aversion to cold, fever, absence of sweating, etc. It is commonly used in the combination with the fresh ginger.

## 201. 鸡苏[1](水苏)

(一)一名水苏。熟捣生叶,绵裹塞耳,疗聋。

(二)又,头风目眩者,以清酒煮汁一升服。产后中风,服之弥佳。

(三)可烧作灰汁及以煮汁洗头,令发香,白屑不生。

(四)又,收讫酿酒及渍酒,常服之佳。

【注释】

[1]鸡苏:又名"水苏"。叶辛香,可以烹鸡,故名。味辛性微温,入肺、脾经,疏风下气,理血辟恶。

## 201. Jisu[1] (Shuisu) [鸡苏 (水苏),
## Chinese fieldnettle, Stachydis Baicalensis Herba]

It is also known as Shuisu. To treat deafness, smash its fresh leaves, wrap them in Mian [绵, silk floss, Bombycis Lana] and put them in the ears.

To treat the people with dizzy vision due to the head wind, decoct 1 Sheng of its juice with the clear liquor and take it. It is especially effective in treating the postpartum wind strike.

Burn it to ash and drench the ash to get ash juice, or decoct it to get juice. Washing hair with the juice can make hair smell fragrant without white dandruff.

After harvesting it, make it into liquor or soak it in liquor. Frequent taking the liquor can achieve desirable effects.

【Note】

[1] Jisu: Also known as Shuisu. With acridity and aroma, its leaves can be used to cook chicken (鸡 in Chinese), for that reason it is called Jisu. Pungent in taste and slightly warm in property, it enters the lung and spleen channel, effective in coursing wind and lowering qi, rectifying the blood and preventing the severe pathogenic factors.

## 202. 香菜[1] (香薷) 温

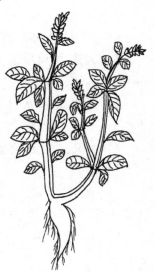

(一) 又云香戎。去热风。生菜中食, 不可多食。

(二) 卒转筋, 可煮汁顿服半升, 止。

(三) 又, 干末止鼻衄, 以水服之。

【注释】

[1] 香菜: 唇形科、香薷属植物, 味辛甘, 性温, 无毒, 发汗解表, 和中利湿, 用于暑湿感冒、恶寒发热、头痛无汗、腹痛吐泻、小便不利。

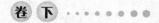

## 202. Xiangrou[1]（Xiangru）［香菜（香薷），mosla, Moslae Herba］ *warm*

It is also known as Xiangrong（香戎）. It can eliminate the heat wind. The fresh Xiangrou（Xiangru）［香菜（香薷），mosla, Moslae Herba］is edible, but do not take it excessively.

To treat the sudden spasm, decoct it and take half a Sheng one time, and the spam will be relieved.

Taking its dry powder with water can treat epistaxis.

【Note】

［1］Xiangrou：The genus of the Lamiaceae of Elsholtzia. Pungent and sweet in taste and mild and non-toxic in property, it can induce sweating to relieve exterior, harmonize the middle and excrete the dampness. It is used to treat the cold due to the summerheat dampness, the aversion to cold with fever, the headache without sweating, the abdominal pain with vomiting and diarrhea and inhibited urination.

## 203. 薄荷 平

解劳。与薤相宜。发汗，通利关节。杵汁服，去心藏风热。

## 203. Bohe［薄荷, peppermint, Herba Menthae］ *mild*

It can relieve fatigue. It is suitable to take it in combination with Xie［薤, Chinese chive, Allii Macrostemonis Bulbus］. It can induce sweating and disinhibit the joints. Taking the juice extracted from crushing it can eliminate the wind heat in the heart.

## 204. 秦荻梨[1]

（一）于生菜中最香美，甚破气。

（二）又，末之，和酒服，疗卒心痛，悒悒，塞满气。

（三）又,子:末以和醋封肿气,日三易。

【注释】

[1] 秦荻梨:味辛,温,无毒,主心腹冷胀,下气,消食。

## 204. Qindili[1][秦荻梨, Qindili medicinal, Materia Medica Qindili]

It has the best fragrance among all the fresh vegetables, and is very effective in breaking the stagnated qi.

To treat the sudden pain in the heart, anxiety and the qi stagnation, grind it into powder and take the powder with liquor.

To treat swelling, grind its seeds into powder, mix them with vinegar before applying them to the swelling, and change them for three times one day.

【Note】

[1] Qindili: Pungent in taste and mild and non-toxic in property, it is mainly used to treat the cold and distention in the heart region and abdomen, break qi stagnation and promote digestion.

## 205. 瓠子[1] 冷

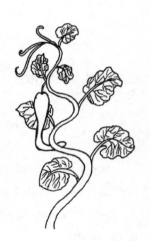

（一）右主治消渴。患恶疮,患脚气虚肿者,不得食之,加甚。

（二）案经:治热风,及服丹石人始可食之。除此,一切人不可食也。患冷气人食之,加甚。又发痼疾。

【注释】

[1] 瓠子:葫芦科葫芦属下的一种,为本属植物葫芦的变种,一年生攀援草本,味甘,性平,有利水、清热、除烦、止渴之功效。

## 205. Huzi[1][瓠子, pericarp of hispid bottle gourd, Lagenariae Clavatae Fructus] *cold*

It is mainly used to treat the consumptive thirst. The people suffering from malign sores and generalized puffy swelling due to the leg qi should not take it as it will exacerbate these symptoms.

The following is supplemented by Zhang Ding：It can treat the wind heat. It is not edible，with the people taking Danshi as the only exception. People suffering from cold qi will get severer illness after eating it. Additionally，it will cause intractable diseases.

**【Note】**

［1］Huzi：The genus of the Cucurbitaceae，a variation of Hulu［葫芦，bottle gourd，Lagenariae Depressae Fructus］，a type of annual herbaceous climbing plant. Sweet in taste and mild in property，it is effective in disinhibiting water，clearing heat，expelling vexation and relieving thirst.

# 206. 大蒜（葫）热

（一）除风,杀虫、毒气。

（二）久服损眼伤肝。治蛇咬疮,取蒜去皮一升,捣以小便一升,煮三、四沸,通人即入溃损处,从夕至暮。初被咬未肿,速嚼蒜封之,六、七易。

（三）又,蒜一升去皮,以乳二升,煮使烂。空腹顿服之,随后饭压之。明日依前进服,下一切冷毒风气。

（四）又,独头者一枚,和雄黄、杏人研为丸,空腹饮下三丸,静坐少时,患鬼气者,当汗出即瘥。

## 206. Dasuan（Hu）［大蒜（葫），garlic，Allii Sativi Bulbus］ *hot*

It can disperse the wind toxin，kill worms and remove the toxic qi.

The long-term taking of it can harm vision and damage the liver. When treating the sores caused by the snakebite，peel 1 Sheng of Dasuan［大蒜，garlic，Allii Sativi Bulbus］，mash it with 1 Sheng of urine，boil them for three or four times. When the decoction's temperature is appropriate，soak the sores into it from afternoon to evening. When just bitten by the snake，chew it quickly，apply it to the affected area and repeat the above procedures for six or seven times before the area is swollen.

Peel 1 Sheng of Dasuan, boil them with 2 Sheng of milk until they are tender, take them at a time before meals, and then have a meal to suppress its taste. Repeating the above procedures the next day will resolve all cold toxin and wind qi then.

When suffering from the ghost qi, grind one Dutousuan〔独头蒜, garlic Allii Sativi Bulbus〕with Xionghuang〔雄黄, realgar, Realgar〕and Xingren〔杏仁, apricot kernel, Armeniacae Semen〕, make pills, take three pills with rice soup before meals, sit down quietly for a while, and then recover after sweating.

# 207. 小蒜(蒜)

（一）主霍乱,消谷,治胃温中,除邪气。五月五日采者上。

（二）又,去诸虫毒、丁肿、毒疮,甚良。不可常食。

## 207. Xiaosuan（Suan）〔小蒜(蒜), scorodoprasum, Allii Scorodoprasi Bulbus〕

It can mainly treat cholera, promote the digestion of food, harmonize the stomach, warm the middle and dispel the evil qi. Xiaosuan〔小蒜, scorodoprasum, Allii Scorodoprasi Bulbus〕, collected on the 5th of the fifth lunar month, can be most effective.

It is also effective in resolving the worm toxin and treating clove sores and toxin sores. It cannot be eaten often.

# 208. 胡　葱 平

（一）主消谷,能食。久食之,令人多忘。根:发痼疾。

（二）又,食著诸毒肉,吐血不止,痿黄悴者:取子一升洗,煮使破,取汁停冷。服半升,日一服,夜一服,血定止。

（三）又,患胡臭[1]、䘌齿人不可食,转极甚。

（四）谨按:利五藏不足气,亦伤绝血脉气。多食损神,此是熏物耳。

【注释】

[1] 胡臭:狐臭。

## 208. Hucong〔胡葱, shallot, Allii Ascalonici Bulbus〕*mild*

It can mainly promote the digestion of food and increase the appetite. The long-term taking of it will cause amnesia. Its roots can cause the chronic diseases.

When suffering from the hematemesis, sallow complexion and haggardness caused by the poisonous meat, wash 1 Sheng of its seeds, boil them in water until they crack, cool the decoction and take half a Sheng of the decoction once during the day and once at night. Stop taking it when the bleeding has been ceased.

It is not suitable for those suffering from the body odor[1] and dental caries for fear that they will get worse.

The following is supplemented by Zhang Ding: It can supplement insufficient qi in the five zang-organs, but can damage and exhaust the blood and qi. The excessive eating of it will damage the spirit, because it is a herb with pungent smell.

**【Note】**

[1] body odor: bromhidrosis.

# 209. 莼 菜

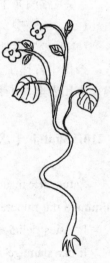

(一) 和鲫鱼作羹,下气止呕。多食动痔。虽冷而补。热食之,亦拥气不下。甚损人胃及齿,不可多食,令人颜色恶。

(二) 又,不宜和醋食之,令人骨痿[1]。少食,补大小肠虚气。久食损毛发。

**【注释】**

[1] 骨痿:肾痿,主要症状有腰背酸软、无法直立、下肢肌肉萎缩松弛、面色暗黑、牙齿干枯。

## 209. Chuncai〔莼菜, water shield, Braseniae Caulis et Folium〕

It can direct qi downward and relieve vomiting by boiling it into the thick soup with Jiyu〔鲫鱼, crucian carp, Carassii Aurati Caro〕and taking the soup. The excessive eating of it can cause hemorrhoids. It is cold in property, but can be used for tonifying and replenishing. Eating it hot will cause the qi stagnation. It can severely damage the stomach and teeth. It is not advisable to eat more as it will make people look pale.

It will also cause the bone wilting[1] when eating it together with vinegar. A small amount of it can supplement the insufficiency of qi in the intestines. The long-term taking of it will damage the hair.

【Note】

〔1〕bone wilting: It is characterized by the weakness of the waist and knees, the inability to stand up, the muscle atrophy of the lower extremities, the loss of facial luster and dry teeth.

## 210. 水 芹 寒

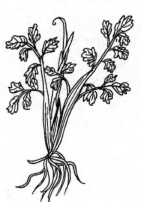

（一）（食之）养神益力,令人肥健。杀石药毒。

（二）置酒酱中香美。

（三）于醋中食之,损人齿,黑色。

（四）生黑滑地,名曰"水芹",食之不如高田者宜人。余田中皆诸虫子在其叶下,视之不见,食之与人为患。高田者名"白芹"。

## 210. Shuiqin〔水芹, water dropwort, Oenanthes Javanicae Herba〕*cold*

Eating it can nourish the spirit, replenish qi and strengthen the body. It can eliminate the mineral intoxication.

It tastes delicious when mixing with liquor or sauce.

It can damage and blacken the teeth when eating it with vinegar.

It grows on the moist low-lying black soil, and is less beneficial to the body health than the one growing in the field of the elevated terrain. Those growing in other fields have small worms beneath their leaves, which are invisible to the human eyes, and they will do harm to the body health after eating them. Those

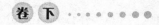

growing in the fields of the elevated terrain are called Baiqin（白芹）.

# 211. 马齿苋

（一）延年益寿，明目。

（二）又，主马毒疮，以水煮，冷服一升，并涂疮上。

（三）患湿癣白秃，取马齿膏涂之。若烧灰敷之，亦良。

（四）作膏：主三十六种风，可取马齿（苋）一硕，水可二硕，蜡三两。煎之成膏。

（五）治疳痢[1]及一切风，敷杖疮良。

（六）及煮一碗，和盐、醋等空腹食之，少时当出尽白虫矣。

（七）又可细切煮粥，止痢，治腹痛。

**【注释】**

[1] 疳痢：小儿疳疾合并痢疾。多因饮食不洁、寒温失调所致。

## 211. Machixian［马齿苋, purslane herb, Herba Portulacae］

It can prolong life and improve vision.

It can also treat the toxin sores of horses by boiling it in water, cooling it, feeding the horses with 1 Sheng of the decoction and applying the decoction to the sores at the same time.

When suffering from the damp lichen and the white bald scalp sore, smear the affected area with its decoction. It is also effective to burn it into ash and apply the ash to the area.

Making paste：Decoct 1 Dan of Machixian［马齿苋, purslane herb, Herba Portulacae］, 2 Dan of water and 3 Liang of wax into paste and the paste can mainly treat thirty-six kinds of wind evils.

It can treat the infantile malnutrition complicated by dysentery[1] and all the diseases caused by the wind evil. It can also treat the injury caused by bludgeoning by applying it to the affected area.

Boil one bowl of Machixian［马齿苋, purslane herb, Herba Portulacae］ with salt and vinegar, take the decoction before meals and the tapeworms will be removed after a short while.

It can relieve dysentery and treat the abdominal pain by chopping it finely and making soup.

【Note】

［1］ infantile malnutrition complicated by dysentery：Infantile malnutrition develops in the course of dysentery，which is mostly caused by the unclean food and the disharmony of cold and warm.

## 212. 落苏（茄子）平

（一）主寒热，五藏劳。不可多食。动气，亦发痼疾。熟者少食之，无畏。患冷人不可食，发痼疾。

（二）又，根：主冻脚疮，煮汤浸之。

（三）又，醋摩之，敷肿毒。

## 212. Luosu（Qiezi）［落苏（茄子），eggplant，Solani Melongenae Fructus］*mild*

It can mainly treat the cold heat and the consumptive disease in the five zang-organs. It is not advisable to eat more, for it will stir qi and cause the intractable diseases. It is fine to take the cooked one a little. People suffering from cold qi can not eat it for fear that it will cause intractable diseases.

Its roots can also mainly treat the foot chilblain by boiling them in water and soaking feet in the water.

It can treat swelling and toxin by grinding its roots with vinegar and applying them to the affected area.

## 213. 蘩蒌

（一）不用令人长食之，恐血尽。或云：蘩蒌即藤也，人恐白软草是。

（二）又方，（治隐轸疮），捣蘩蒌封上。

（三）煮作羹食之，甚益人。

### 213. Fanlou〔蘩蒌, malachium, Stellariae Herba〕

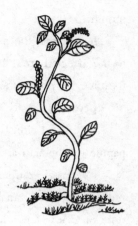

It is not advisable to eat it for a long time for fear that it may exhaust blood. Some people say that it is a kind of vine, while others say it is Bairuancao（白软草）.

It can also treat urticaria by mashing and applying it to the affected area.

It can nourish the human body by boiling it into thick soup and taking the soup.

### 214. 鸡肠草 温

（一）作灰和盐,疗一切疮及风丹[1]遍身如枣大、痒痛者:捣封上,日五、六易之。

（二）亦可生食,煮作菜食之,益人。去脂膏毒气。

（三）治一切恶疮,捣汁傅之,五月五日者验。

（四）又,烧傅疳䘌[2]。亦疗小儿赤白痢,可取汁一合,和蜜服之甚良。

【注释】

[1] 风丹:病症名,症见皮肤有斑疹隐隐显露、瘙痒、皮色不红。

[2] 疳䘌:鼻前庭炎,多伴有疼痛、发热干燥等临床症状。另见 83 条"沙糖"注释 2。

### 214. Jichangcao〔鸡肠草, malachium, Stellariae Herba〕 *warm*

It can treat all the sores, the wind cinnabar[1] as big as a jujube all over the body, the itching and pain by burning it into ash and mixing the ash with salt. Mash and apply it to the affected area for five or six times a day.

Both cooked and uncooked Jichangcao〔鸡肠草, malachium, Stellariae Herba〕can nourish the human body. It can remove the toxicity of fat.

It can treat all the severe sores by mashing it and applying its juice to the affected area, and it will be more effective if collected on the 5th of the fifth lunar month.

It can treat the nasal vestibulitis[2] by burning it into ash and applying the ash to the affected area. It can also treat the red and white dysentery by mixing 1 Ge of its juice with honey and taking the juice.

【Notes】

［1］wind cinnabar: It is a disease characterized by the faintly visible macula and papule on the skin and itching without the skin turning red.

［2］nasal vestibulitis: It is a disease characterized by the chronic and recurrent redness, swelling, anabrosis, crust and itching of the nasal vestibule. See the second note of Clause 83 "Shatang 沙糖".

## 215. 白 苣 寒

（一）主补筋力。

（二）利五藏,开胸膈拥塞气,通经脉,养筋骨,令人齿白净,聪明,少睡。可常常食之。有小冷气人食之,虽亦觉腹冷,终不损人。

（三）又,产后不可食之,令人寒中[1],少腹痛。

（四）味苦寒一云平。主补筋骨,利五脏,开胸膈拥气,通经脉,止脾气。令人齿白,聪明,少睡。可常食之。患冷气人食,即腹冷,不至苦损人。产后不可食,令人寒中,小腹痛。

【注释】

［1］寒中:病症名,指邪在脾胃而见里寒的病症。

### 215. Baiju ［白苣, lettuce, Lactucae Sativae Caulis et Folium］*cold*

It can mainly strengthen the sinews and bones and increase energy.

It can harmonize the five zang-organs, disperse qi stagnation in the chest and diaphragm, dredge collaterals, strengthen the sinews and bones, whiten the teeth, improve hearing and vision and reduce fatigue. It is advisable to eat it often. Those suffering from slight cold qi will feel cold in the abdomen after eating it, but that will not damage the body health.

It is not advisable to eat it after the delivery of a baby, for it will cause the cold parapoplexy[1] and slight abdominal pain.

It is pungent in taste and cold in property, while some people say that it is mild in property. It can mainly strengthen the sinews and bones, harmonize the five zang-organs, disperse qi stagnation in the chest and diaphragm, dredge collaterals and balance spleen qi. It can whiten the teeth, improve hearing and vision and reduce fatigue. It is advisable to eat it often. Those suffering from cold qi will feel cold in the abdomen after eating it, but that will not damage the body health. It is not advisable to eat it after the delivery of a baby, for it will cause the cold parapoplexy and slight abdominal pain.

【Note】

[1] cold parapoplexy: It is a syndrome caused by the interior cold due to the pathogen in the spleen and stomach.

# 216. 落 葵

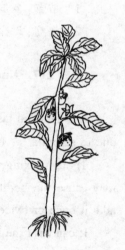

（一）其子悦泽人面，药中可用之。

（二）其子令人面鲜华可爱。取蒸，烈日中曝干。按去皮，取人细研，和白蜜敷之，甚验。

（三）食此菜后被狗咬，即疮不瘥也。

## 216. Luokui〔落葵, Malabar spinach,
### Basellae Rubrae Folium seu Herba〕

Its seeds can moisturize the facial skin and can be used in the beauty prescriptions.

Its seeds can make the facial skin delicate and glowing. It will be particularly effective to steam its seeds, expose them to the blazing sun, rub their skins to get kernels, grind the kernels, mix the powder with honey and smear the face with that.

The wounds will not heal easily if bitten by dogs after eating it.

# 217. 堇 菜[1]

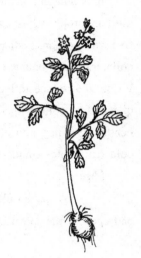

（一）味苦。主寒热鼠瘘，瘰疬[2]生疮，结核聚气。下瘀血。

（二）久食，除心烦热，令人身重懈惰。又令人多睡，只可一两顿而已。

（三）又，捣敷热肿良。

（四）又，杀鬼毒，生取汁半升服，即吐出。

（五）叶：主霍乱。与香薷同功。蛇咬：生研敷之，毒即出矣。

（六）又，干末和油煎成，摩结核上，三、五度便瘥。

【注释】

[1] 堇菜：多年生草本，性寒，味微苦，有清热解毒之功效。

[2] 瘰疬：又称"老鼠疮"，是生于颈部的一种感染性外科疾病。

## 217. Jincai[1]〔堇菜，violet，Violae Formosanae Herba〕

It is bitter in taste. It can treat the cold and heat, the mouse fistula, the sores due to scrofula[2], tuberculosis and qi stagnation and eliminate the static blood.

Though taking it often can eliminate the heat vexation in the heart, this diet may cause the bodily heaviness, laziness and somnolence. So people had better take it once or twice occasionally.

It can treat the heat toxic swelling with great effects by externally applying the pounded one on the affected part.

It can kill the ghost toxin and help spit out the ghost toxin by taking half a Sheng of the pounded juice of it.

Its leaves can treat cholera, which has the same effect as Xiangru〔香薷，mosla, Moslae Herba〕does. It can treat the snake bites and dispel the venom out by applying the ground fresh one externally to the wounds.

It can cure the tuberculosis by applying the oily-fried paste of the powder ground out of the dry one to the tuberculosis three to five times.

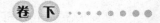

【Note】

[1] Jincai: A perennial herb, slightly bitter in taste and cold in property, has the effects of clearing heat and removing toxin.

[2] scrofula: Also known as mouse sores, an infectious surgical disease in people's neck.

## 218. 蕺菜（鱼腥草）[1] 温

小儿食之,便觉脚痛,三岁不行。久食之,发虚弱,损阳气,消精髓,不可食。

【注释】

[1] 蕺菜:腥臭草本植物,有异味。全株入药,有清热、解毒、利水之功效。

## 218. Jicai[1] (Yuxingcao) [蕺菜（鱼腥草）, houttuynia, Houttuyniae Herba] *warm*

The children who take it may get sore feet, thus they cannot walk until they are three years old. It should not be taken for a long time, because it may cause the vacuity disease, impair the yang qi and consume the essence-marrow.

【Note】

[1] Jicai: A stinky herb which has a peculiar smell. The whole plant can be used as drug and it has the effects of clearing heat, removing toxin and disinhibiting water.

## 219. 马芹子[1]

和酱食诸味良。根及叶不堪食。卒心痛:子作末,醋服。

【注释】

[1] 马芹子:孜然,是常用的调味品,味辛,性温,有散寒止痛、理气宽中之功效。

### 219. Maqinzi[1]〔马芹子, cumin, Cuminum Cyminum〕

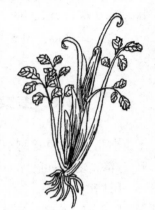

It tastes good when mixed with sauces. Its roots and leaves should not be taken. It can treat the sudden heart pain by taking its ground powder with vinegar.

**【Note】**

[1] Maqinzi: The cumin, which is a common seasoning. It is pungent in taste and mild in property and has the effects of dispersing cold, relieving pain, regulating qi and smoothing the middle.

## 220. 芸苔(油菜)[1]

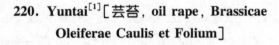

（一）若先患腰膝,不可多食,必加极。
（二）又,极损阳气,发口疮,齿痛。
（三）又,能生腹中诸虫。道家特忌。

**【注释】**

[1] 芸苔:别名油菜花,二年生草本植物,叶可食,有散血消肿之功效。

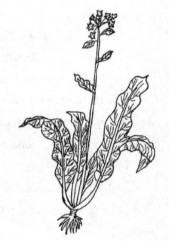

### 220. Yuntai[1]〔芸苔, oil rape, Brassicae Oleiferae Caulis et Folium〕

It should not be taken too much by the people who have already got the disease of the lumbus and knees because it may worsen the disease.

It impairs yang qi greatly and causes the mouth ulcers and toothache.

It can also breed many kinds of parasites in the abdomen. Thus the Taoists avoid it as a taboo.

**【Note】**

[1] Yuntai: It is also known as the rape flower, a biennial herb. Its leaves are edible. It has the effects of dissipating the blood stasis and dispersing swelling.

## 221. 雍 菜[1]

（一）味甘，平，无毒。主解野葛毒，煮食之。亦生捣服之。岭南种之。蔓生，花白，堪为菜。云南人先食雍菜，后食野葛，二物相伏，自然无苦。

（二）又，取汁滴野葛苗，当时烟死，其相杀如此。张司空云：魏武帝啖野葛至一尺。应是先食此菜也。

**【注释】**

［1］雍菜：又名"空心菜"，蔓生植物，喜高温多湿环境，有清热解毒之功效。

## 221. Yongcai[1]［雍菜，water spinach，Ipomoeae Aquaticae Caulis et Folium］

It is sweet in taste and mild and non-toxic in property. It can remove the toxin of Yege［野葛，yellow jessamine，Gelsemii Herba］by taking the boiled one or its pounded juice. It grows in Lingnan, trailing over the ground with white flowers and can be taken as vegetable. The people in Yunnan prefer to take it first and Yege［野葛，yellow jessamine，Gelsemii Herba］later, because these two foods are mutually restricted to each other thus taking them both can relieve the harm.

Dropping its juice onto the shoots of Yege［野葛，yellow jessamine，Gelsemii Herba］can make the latter one wither to death on the spot, which can obviously demonstrate the degree of their hostility to each other. Zhang Sikong said, "Emperor Wu of Wei can take 1 Chi of Yege［野葛，yellow jessamine，Gelsemii Herba］each meal without getting harms, and he must have taken it first."

**【Note】**

［1］Yongcai：It is also known as Kongxincai, a trailing plant. It prefers the hot and wet living environment and has the effects of clearing heat and removing toxin.

## 222. 菠薐[1]（菠菜）

冷，微毒。利五藏，通肠胃热，解酒毒。服丹石人食之佳。北人食肉面即平，南人食鱼鳖水米即冷。不可多食，冷大小肠。久食令人脚弱不能行。发腰痛，不与蛆鱼同食。发霍乱吐泻。

【注释】

[1] 菠薐:菠菜,一年生草本植物,是极常见的蔬菜之一,有养血、止血、敛阴、润燥之功效。

## 222. Boleng[1] (Bocai) [菠薐(菠菜), spinach, Spinaciae Herba cum Radice]

It is cold and slightly toxic in property. It can tonify and replenish the five zang-organs, clear the evil heat in the stomach and intestines and resolve the liquor toxin. It is very good to the people who take Danshi. It is mild in property to the northerners who often take meat and wheaten food while it is cold in property to the southerners who often take fish, turtles and rice. It should not be taken too much, because it may make the large and small intestines catch cold. Neither should be taken often, because it may weaken the feet and legs, causing inability to walk. It should not be taken with mud eels, it will otherwise cause lumbago. It can cause cholera, vomiting and diarrhea.

【Note】

[1] Boleng: It is also called Bocai, an annual herb, one of the most common vegetables. It has the effects of nourishing blood, stopping bleeding, constraining yin and moistening dryness.

# 223. 苦荬[1]

冷,无毒。治面目黄,强力,止困,敷蛇虫咬。又,汁敷丁肿,即根出。蚕蛾出时,切不可取拗,令蛾子青烂。蚕妇亦忌食。野苦荬五六回拗后,味甘滑于家苦荬,甚佳。

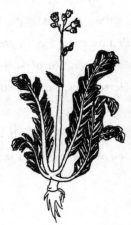

【注释】

[1] 苦荬:别名"苦菜",多年生草本,可做蔬菜食用,有清热解毒、消痈排脓、祛瘀止痛之功效。

## 223. Kumai[1] [苦荬, denticulate ixeris,
## Ixeris Denticulatae Herba]

It is cold and non-toxic in property. It can treat the yellow face, increase strength, relieve drowsiness. It can treat the snake bite and the worm bite by applying it externally. It can remove the toxic qi from the root of the swelling of clove sores by applying its juice externally. It should not be picked when the silk moths get out of their cocoons, because its toxin can make the silk moths putrefied. So those women who raise silk moths should not take it. The wild one, after picked several times, will taste sweeter and more delicate than those growing in the garden.

**【Note】**

[1] Kumai: It is also called Kucai [苦菜, bitter sow thistle, Sonchi Oleracei Herba], a perennial herb, which can be taken as vegetable. It has the effects of clearing heat and removing toxin, dispersing welling-abscesses and expelling pus, dispelling stasis and relieving pains.

## 224. 鹿角菜[1]

大寒,无毒,微毒。下热风气,疗小儿骨蒸热劳。丈夫不可久食,发痼疾,损经络血气,令人脚冷痹,损腰肾,少颜色。服丹石人食之,下石力也。出海州,登、莱沂、密州并有,生海中。又能解面热。

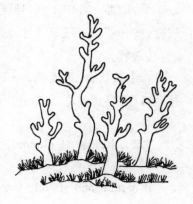

**【注释】**

[1] 鹿角菜:杉藻科角叉菜属藻体,是一种重要经济海藻,具有软坚散结、清热解毒、和胃通便等功效。

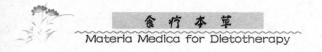

### 224. Lujiaocai[1]〔鹿角菜，glue plant，Gloiopeltis〕

It is severely cold, non-toxic or slightly toxic in property. It can disperse the heat evil and the wind evil and treat children's steaming bone fever. The men should not take it for a long time, because it may cause the intractable disease, impair collaterals, qi and blood, cause cold and impediment pain of the feet and legs, impair the lumbar and kidney and make the complexion bad. Those who take Danshi should not take it either, because it may reduce the effect of Danshi. It grows in the regions such as Haizhou, Dengzhou, Laizhou, Yizhou and Mizhou. It grows in the seawater and can remove the heat of wheaten food.

【Note】

[1] Lujiaocai：An algae which belongs to the Chondrus Stackhouse of the Genus Gigartinaceae. It is one of the important economic algas and has the effects of softening hardness and dissipating mass, clearing heat and removing toxin, harmonizing the stomach and freeing stool.

## 225. 莙荙[1]（甜菜）

平,微毒。补中下气,理脾气,去头风,利五藏。冷气不可多食,动气。先患腹冷,食必破腹。茎灰淋汁,洗衣白如玉色。

【注释】

[1] 莙荙:叶用甜菜,一年生或二年生草本叶菜,嫩叶可做蔬菜食用,有清热解毒、行瘀止血之功效。

### 225. Junda[1]（Tiancai）〔莙荙（甜菜），lycium leaf，Lycii Folium〕

It is mild and slightly toxic in property. It can tonify the middle, lower qi, regulate the spleen qi, relieve the recurrent headache, tonify and replenish the five zang-oragans. Those who suffer from cold qi should not take it, because it may stir qi. Those who suffer from cold abdomen should not take it either, because it will definitely cause the frequent diarrhea. It can wash clothes as white as a polished jade by using the water of burnt stem ash.

**【Note】**

［1］Junda：Spinach beet, an annual or biennial herb. Its fresh leaves can make dishes. It has the effects of clearing heat and removing toxin, resolving stasis and stopping bleeding.

## 226. 附 馀[1]

孟诜方:治产后血运心闷气绝方

以冷水噀面即醒。

孟诜食经方:鱼骨哽方

取萩去皮,着鼻中,少时瘥。

孟诜食经云:拧茎单煮洗浴之。

又方,茺蔚[2]可作浴汤。

又方,煮赤小豆取汁停冷洗,不过三四。

又方,捣蘩蒌封上。

白鸽肉:"诜曰暖"。

"调精益气,治恶疮疥癣,风疮白癜,疬疡风。炒熟酒服,虽益人,食多恐减药力。孟诜。"

**【注释】**

［1］附馀:这部分均为《医心方》直接引用《食疗本草》的佚文。

［2］茺蔚:益母草,一年或二年生草本,有活血、祛淤、调经、消水之功效。

## 226. Extras[1]

Meng Shen：Therapy to treat the postpartum syncope due to the blood dizziness, vexation and oppression.

Spraying the cold water to the faces of women who have just given birth can make them gain consciousness.

Meng Shen's *Shi Liao Ben Cao* [《食疗本草》, *Materia Medica for Dietotherapy*]：Therapy to treat the fish bones stuck in the throat.

Peel the skin of the wormwood and put it into the nose. A little while later, the fish bone will go out.

Meng Shen's *Shi Liao Ben Cao* [《食疗本草》, *Materia Medica for Dietotherapy*] records: Boil the stems alone and use the water to bathe.

Chongwei[2] [茺蔚, leonurus, Leonuri Herba] can be made as the decoction for bath.

The cool decoction of Chixiaodou [赤小豆, rice bean, Phaseoli Semen] can be used to bathe three or four times.

Use the pounded Fanlou [繁蒌, Chickweed, Stellaria media] to seal.

The pigeon meat: Meng Shen said it was warm in property.

It can regulate essence, replenish qi, treat the malign sores, scab, lichen, wind papules, white patch wind and pityriasis versicolor. People can take the fried pigeon meat with liquor. Though it can tonify and replenish the body, people should not take too much of it, because it may reduce the drug effect. Meng Shen.

**【Notes】**

[1] Extras: This part is the direct quotation of the lost writings of *Shi Liao Ben Cao* [《食疗本草》, *Materia Medica for Dietotherapy*] from *Yi Xin Fang* [《医心方》, *Formula from the Heart of Physicians*].

[2] Chongwei: It is also known as Yimucao, an annual or biennial herb, which has the effects of activating blood, resolving stasis, regulating menstruation and dispersing the water swelling.